STUDIES IN THE HISTORY OF OPHTHALMOLOGY IN ENGLAND

PLATE I

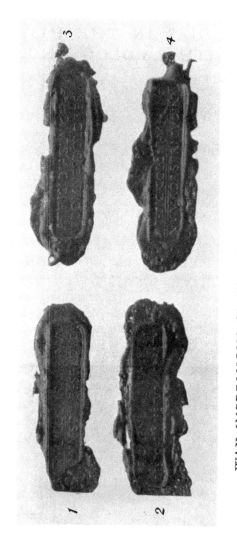

WAX IMPRESSIONS OF THE CIRENCESTER (2) STAMP

First published by kind permission of Mrs Wilfred Cripps

STUDIES IN

THE HISTORY OF OPHTHALMOLOGY
IN ENGLAND

PRIOR TO THE YEAR 1800

by

R. RUTSON JAMES, F.R.C.S.Eng.

Consulting Ophthalmic Surgeon to St George's Hospital and
Senior Editor of the British Journal of Ophthalmology

Let us now praise famous men, and our fathers
that begat us.   ECCLESIASTICUS XLIV. I

Inventas aut qui vitam excoluere per artis,
Quique sui memores alios fecere merendo.
VIRGIL, *Aeneid* VI

CAMBRIDGE
AT THE UNIVERSITY PRESS
Published for
The British Journal of Ophthalmology
1933

CAMBRIDGE UNIVERSITY PRESS
Cambridge, New York, Melbourne, Madrid, Cape Town,
Singapore, São Paulo, Delhi, Mexico City

Cambridge University Press
The Edinburgh Building, Cambridge CB2 8RU, UK

Published in the United States of America by Cambridge University Press, New York

www.cambridge.org
Information on this title: www.cambridge.org/9781107625495

© Cambridge University Press 1933

First published 1933
First paperback edition 2013

A catalogue record for this publication is available from the British Library

ISBN 978-1-107-62549-5 Paperback

CONTENTS

PLATES

PREFACE

IN the following pages an attempt is made to trace some phases of the history of ophthalmology in England from the earliest times to the end of the eighteenth century.

Much of the contents does not now appear for the first time. During the past nine years, in which I have been a member of the editorial staff of the *British Journal of Ophthalmology*, I have contributed to that journal, and to some others, numerous papers of a biographical and quasi-historical nature. For the most part these papers have undergone abstraction in this book; some, *e.g.* those on Anglo-Saxon Ophthalmology, Turberville of Salisbury and William Briggs are here presented almost as they were first printed.

I am under an obligation to Sir John Parsons, F.R.S., the Chairman, and to the other members of the editorial committee, for encouragement, permission to utilise the articles which have appeared in the journal, and for the loan of blocks for illustration. I have permission to reprint the historical papers by the late George Coats, F.R.C.S., which are contained in the last volume of the Moorfields Reports. It was felt to be a pity that these biographical papers of the first class, by one who was a dear friend to many of us, should not have a wider circulation than was possible in their original setting. And so it was determined to include them. Coats's paper on the Chevalier's grandson oversteps my limit of the end of the eighteenth century, but it was thought best to reproduce them in their entirety. I am afraid that many of the chapters are superficial. They do not claim to be exhaustive; and I plead guilty to having neglected the subject of optics after the thirteenth century. Those of my readers who expected to find more detail on optics than is contained here must be content to:

> "Doat with Copernicus, or darkling stray
> With *Bacon*, Ptolemy, or Tycho Brahe!"

to make a small variation in the couplet from "Architectural Atoms" in the *Rejected Addresses*.

I have to record my grateful thanks to my friends Mr Duke-Elder, Dr Ernest Thomson, of Stirling, and Mr Arnold Sorsby. The former read the manuscript, gave me the benefit of his criticism and has helped in correcting the proofs; Dr Thomson has read the proofs also and has polished my rough prose; while Mr Sorsby has kindly allowed me to abstract his valuable paper on Milton's blindness, and those on the books of Richard Banister, "A.H." and Sir William Read. To him I also owe my acquaintance with the little book by Robert Turner.

My heaviest debt of gratitude is due to Mr J. Harvey Bloom for undertaking the necessary research at the British Museum, at the Public Record Office and at Somerset House. My knowledge of the important MS. in the Sloane Collection is entirely due to him, and I am glad to testify to the advantages this book has derived from the work of so experienced an authority on records and record-searching.

Finally, I must record my indebtedness to the members of the Library staff of the Royal College of Surgeons of England and the Royal Society of Medicine, and to the Cambridge University Press for the care they have taken. All the blocks for illustration with two exceptions have been made by Messrs George Pulman and Sons of Thayer St., Manchester Square.

I hope that some English surgeon may be tempted to complete the work by adding a volume, later, on the giants of the nineteenth century.

R. R. JAMES

46 WIMPOLE STREET
W. I.

CHAPTER I

Ophthalmology in Roman Britain

THE dawn of ophthalmology in Britain dates from the Roman occupation. Prior to this time we have no records, and apart from charms and the belief in the evil eye, which are of immense antiquity, and have nothing to do with ophthalmology in the accepted meaning of the term, we can only assume that as Britain was inhabited, diseases of the eye must have existed from the earliest times; and we can imagine neolithic man sitting down to flake his flints and occasionally receiving a corneal abrasion, or a perforating injury. It may also be permissible to guess that, as our forbears coloured themselves with woad, they must have possessed some degree of colour vision. Whether the different tribes used a universal tint, or whether variation was allowed, we do not know, but I have always liked to think that the shade of colour of *e.g.* the Brigantes in the North may have been different from that of the Iceni in East Anglia, and from that of the Silures on the Welsh March. But, with the settling of Britain as a Roman colony, ophthalmology came into being. Diseases of the eye were common in the Roman Empire and a class of practitioners, which undertook their treatment, existed. Galen gathered up the ophthalmic knowledge of his time and speaks, in one of his books, of a "forest" of collyria. According to Sir James Simpson, Galen gives the formulae for about a couple of hundred of these collyria. Some of them achieved so great a reputation that in time they acquired specific names; these were sometimes derived from the name of the original compounder (like Guthrie's hell-fire lotion of the last century). More often the name was derived from some specific property (*chloron*, green; *cirrhon*, yellow; *aromaticum*, from the pleasant odour). The collyrium Diasmyrnes contained myrrh, the Diarrhodon, rose-water;

some were named from their cheapness, others from their great value; finally a collyrium was frequently known under some high-sounding but unmeaning name, such as Olympus, Proteus, Phoenix, etc.

The main evidence we have of ophthalmology in this country in Roman times consists of the numerous examples of Roman oculists' stamps which have been unearthed during the last two centuries. Esperandieu's authoritative *Signacula Medicorum Oculariorum* (1904) gives details of more than two hundred specimens of Roman stamps, and in a paper which I contributed to the *British Journal of Ophthalmology* in March 1926 I was able to describe twenty which have been found in Britain; and since that date I have collected notes of three other examples.

These stamps for the main part agree in their general characteristics. They are usually small quadrilateral or oblong pieces of stone engraved on one or more of their borders. The inscriptions are in small capital Roman letters, cut retrograde and intagliate, and consequently reading on the stone itself from right to left, but making an impression when stamped on wax or other plastic material which reads from left to right. These inscriptions generally first contain (and this is repeated on each side) the name of the practitioner to whom the stamp belonged, then the name of some special medicament, and lastly the disease for which the medicine was prescribed. Occasionally the mode and frequency of using the preparation are added. Two of the stamps unearthed in Britain are peculiar in that they are circular and the inscription is cut on the face. These stamps were probably intended to impress the directions for use on the semi-solid ointment, much as a maker's name is stamped on a modern cake of soap.

Roman stamps have been found at Tranent, in East Lothian; at Gloucester (this stamp was at first falsely designated the Colchester stamp); at Bath; at Littleborough, Notts.; at Wroxeter, Salop; at Kenchester, Herefordshire; at Cirencester (2); in county Tipperary; at Leicester; at Sandy, Beds.; at Colchester; at Lydney, Glos.; at Harrold, Beds.; and at Lansdown, near Bath. One of the recent finds came from near Crediton and the other two from the City of London.

Ireland is usually said not to have been subject to Rome, but Roman antiquities have been found there and among them a stamp* which is now in the British Museum. It is engraved on one side, as follows:

M JUVEN TUTIANI
DIAMYSUS AD VET CIC.

This may be extended, *M. Juventii Tutiani Diamysus ad veteres cicatrices*, and translated "the Diamysus of M. Juventius Tutianus for old scars". Simpson, from whose classical papers I have derived most of my knowledge on this subject and from whom I largely quote, states that the Diamysus derives its name from the fact that the principal ingredient was misy, a metallic vitriolic preparation, useful as a stimulant and escharotic: as late as the year 1662 it still occupied a place in the London Pharmacopœia. According to Adams, misy was a combination of sulphate of copper with sulphate of iron.

As an example of a stamp with greater variety of inscription I may give the Cirencester stamp No. 2, in the museum of the late Mrs Wilfred Cripps. It was dug up in the year 1900, in ground near the G.W.R. station. This is a square stamp, each side measuring $1\frac{3}{4}$ inches in length, the depth being $\frac{1}{4}$ inch. The inscriptions are as follows:

1. ATTICI COLLYR TURINUM
   AD OMNES DOLORES EX OVO.

2. ATTICI LENE AD OMNES DOLO
   RES POST IMPETUM LIPPITU.

3. ATTICI DIAGLAUCAEUM
   AD OMNES DOLORES F.

4. ATTICI COLLYR MELI
   NUM AD ASPRITRUDIN F.

* Perhaps the owner may have been summoned to Ireland from England to treat some great Irish lord and have left his stamp behind him or lost it on the way.

Inscriptions No. 1 and No. 4 have fine parallel lines separating the two halves of lettering; between the lines on the second inscription is the representation of a swastica. I do not know what the letter "F" means in the third and fourth inscriptions. The word *turinum* in the first inscription means frankincense; it was to be used with white of egg in cases of pain. The second inscription may be rendered "the mild application of Atticus for all pain following lippitudo" (either conjunctivitis or blepharitis, or a mixture of the two).

I surmise that the word *diaglaucaeum* may mean the green dialebanum; while the last inscription may be rendered "the *collyrium melinum* of Atticus for granulations". Galen makes mention of the *collyrium melinum*. Opinions differ as to its origin; whether from *malum*, an apple; or from the island of Melos, whence the ancients obtained their alum; or from *melinum*, meaning yellow.

It will be seen that this stamp allows Atticus four different kinds of treatment, one of them to be used with white of egg, by which he can alleviate pain, inflammation and granulations.

Among the Roman stamps of Britain are the circular ones of Wroxeter and Leicester. I feel that doubt may be expressed as to the latter being really a Roman oculist's stamp, but it is included by Deneffe, in his pamphlet *Les Oculistes Gallo-Romains au IIIe Siècle* (1896); it may with equal justice be considered a tradesman's stamp. But no doubt exists as to the Wroxeter stamp, now in the Shrewsbury Museum. This was unearthed in 1808 by a ploughman when ploughing a field near the "old wall". Figured and described by Parkes, in the *Gentleman's Magazine* in 1810, it was also mentioned by Nightingale in his *Beauties of England and Wales*; while Hartshorne, in *Salopia Antiqua* (1841), wrongly described it as an amuletal seal. This description was corrected by Albert Way, by Wright in his *Celt, Roman and Saxon*, and Simpson finally gave the best rendering. The inscription is on the face and is as follows:

IBCLM

DIA LBA

AD OM

NE Δ UN

O EX O.

Simpson has extended this into J(*ulii*) B(*assi*) *Clementis Diale-*
banum ad omnem Διάθεσιν *uno ex ovo*; and has translated it "the
Dialebanum (incense collyrium) of Julius Bassus Clemens for
every disease of the eye, to be used mixed with white of egg".

The stamp has the rude figure of a plant engraved at one side of
the inscription and Hartshorne confused himself and others by
reading this figure as a letter at the beginning of the third line.
Simpson has pointed out that in Roman times the Greek word
diathesis meant the disease itself and not, as nowadays, the
tendency to the disease.

There can be no doubt that practitioners in Britain in Roman
times were well equipped with formulae for ointments to be
used in diseases of the eye. Whether their cirrhon (yellow)
ointment was as popular then as the well-known golden ointment of the last two centuries I cannot say; but the few examples
I have given show a variety of medicaments to be employed for
a variety of disorders. In two instances, among those cited,
impressions of oculists' stamps have been found on jars or pots,
in one case of red Samian ware; one of which was discovered,
appropriately enough, in the neighbourhood of Moorfields Eye
Hospital.

We must be careful, however, not to draw unwarranted con-
clusions from the ingredients of these ointments as to the types
of eye disease present at this remote period; and I do not think
that because a Roman collyrium contained copper, we have any
justification for the belief that trachoma was necessarily endemic
in Britain. There may have been sporadic cases.

I am not aware of any evidence to show that ophthalmic
operations were much practised in Roman Britain. I should
surmise that any eye operations which may have been per-

formed would probably deal with conditions affecting the eyelids, such as ingrowing lashes, rather than the globe itself. Pterygia, if present, may have been cut off and lacrymal fistulae scraped. It is possible that such a malposition of the lid as entropion may have been treated by the very early procedure of cutting away a fold of skin, thereby leading in some instances to gross shortening of the lid. Since the Carthaginians are said to have cut away the eyelids of the Roman general Regulus with great freedom of hand, it may be that a practitioner in this outpost of the Empire occasionally removed the lash-bearing border of the lid in cases of inveterate ingrowing lashes. Cataracts may have been couched.

CHAPTER II

Anglo-Saxon Ophthalmology

OPHTHALMIC LEECHDOMS

IN THE YEARS 1864, 1865, 1866 there were published, in the Rolls Series, three volumes by the Rev. Oswald Cockayne, entitled *Leechdoms, Wortcunning and Starcraft in Early England*. These give the main facts about ophthalmology in Anglo-Saxon times.

The question of continuity in England after the departure of the Romans and before the pacification of the Heptarchy is a much disputed point. Authorities, such as the late Professor Haverfield and Mr Collingwood, are in favour of there being no continuity between the Roman and Saxon epochs. On the other hand, Professor Zachrisson, of Upsala, working on place-name material, holds that "for philological reasons a conscious and artificial revival of Roman names is entirely out of the question".

Mr Cockayne, in his preface, would seem to support the latter tenet. He held that the Saxons accepted Greek and Latin learning, and that the Gothic nations had a knowledge of the kinds and powers of worts, *i.e.* the practical part of botany: "their medicines must have consisted partly in the application of the qualities of these worts to healing purposes, for otherwise the study was of no real utility". Charms played a large part. Marcellus, *c.* A.D. 380, recommends, "to avoid inflamed eyes, when you see a star fall or cross the heavens, count quickly, for you will be free from inflammation for as many years as you count numbers". Chastity on the part of the patient and the leech, coupled with Greek word written on parchment and suspended round the neck, will work wonders. "As soon as a man gets pain in his eyes, tie in unwrought flax as many knots as there are letters in his name, pronouncing them as you go, and tie it round his neck."

"For white spot, as cataract, catch a fox alive; cut his tongue out; let him go; dry his tongue and tie it up in a red rag and hang it round the man's neck. If anything to cause annoyance get into a man's eye, with five fingers of the same side as the eye, run the eye over and fumble at it, saying three times, 'tetunc resonco, bregan gresso', and spit thrice. For the same, shut the vexed eye and say thrice, 'in mon deromarcos axatison', and spit thrice; this remedy is 'mirificum'. For the same, shut the other eye, touch gently the vexed eye with the ring finger and thumb, and say thrice, 'I buss the Gorgons mouth'. For hordeolum, which is a sore place in the eyelid, of the shape of a barleycorn, take nine grains of barley and with each poke the sore, with every one saying the magic words, 'kuria kuria kassaria sourophbi', then throw away the nine, and do the same with seven; throw away seven, and do the same with five, and so with three and one. For the same, take nine grains of barley and poke the sore, and at every poke say 'pheuge pheuge krithe se diokei', 'flee, flee, barley thee chaseth'. For the same, touch the sore with the medicinal or ring finger, and say thrice, 'vigaria gasaria'."

The first of these volumes consists of an Anglo-Saxon *Herbarium*, derived partly from Apuleius and partly from Dioscorides, together with the *Medicina de Quadripedibus* of Sextus Placitus, with some fly-leaf leechdoms and charms. The second volume consists of three leech books; the first two form a treatise on medicine with its proper colophon at the end, the third is of a more monkish character. The book probably belonged to the abbey of Glastonbury. In the colophon is the following, "Bald habet hunc librum Cild quem conscribere jussit". Bald was the owner, Cild, the scribe. The former seems to have been an Anglo-Saxon general practitioner, and he had some knowledge of eye prescriptions.

In volume I, the herbs are arranged in a sort of index, with the conditions for which they are of use. With regard to ophthalmic complaints, these are usually sore eyes, sometimes dimness of sight, occasionally bleared eyes; swelling of the eye is mentioned often, erysipelas once, headache more frequently.

I propose to take the various herbs useful for eye conditions and abstract what is said about them in the body of the work.

BETONY. To be gathered in the month of August, without use of iron; when gathered, shake the mould, till none of it cleave thereon, and then dry it in the shade very thoroughly, and with its roots altogether reduce it to dust; then use, and taste of it when thou needest. For sore of eyes, take the roots of the same wort, seethe them in water to the third part (evaporating two-thirds of the water), and with the water bathe the eyes, and take leaves of the same wort and bruise them and lay them over the eyes upon the face. For dimness of sight take the same root, by weight one drachm, and give (the patient) to drink fasting, then it diminishes the part of the blood from which dimness cometh. For blear eyes, take of the same wort betony, and give (the patient) to swallow, it will do good and will clear the sharpness of the eyes.

MUGWORT (*Artemisia vulgaris*). It turneth away the evil eyes of evil men.

RAVENS LEEK (*Orchis*). For sore of eyes, that is, when that one be tearful, take juice of this same wort, and smear the eyes therewith; without delay it removes the sore.

KNOTGRASS (*Polygonum aviculare*). For sore of eyes, before sunrise, or shortly before it begin fully to set, go to the same wort proserpinaca, and scratch it round about with a golden ring, and say that thou wilt take it for leechdom of eyes, and after three days go again thereto before rising of sun, and take it, and hang it about the man's swere (neck); it will profit well.

MAYTHE (*Anthemis nobilis*). For sore of eyes, let a man take ere the upgoing of the sun..and when he taketh it, let him say that he will take it against white specks, and against sore of eyes; let him take next the ooze and smear the eyes therewith.

WOOD LETTUCE. For dimness of eyes, it is said that the earn (eagle) when he will upfly, in order that he may see the more brightly, will touch his eyes with the juice, and wet them, and he through that obtains the greatest brightness. Again for dimness of eyes, take juice of this same wort, mixed with old wine and with honey, and let this be collected without smoke. It is best that a man mingle together juice of this wort, and wine and honey, and lay them up in a glass ampulla; use when need be; from this you will observe a wondrous cure.

GARCLIVE (*Agrimony*). For sore of eyes, take this wort, which is named agrimony; pound it so green by itself; if then thou have it not green take it dry and dip it in warm water, so as thou may earliest use it; smear then therewith; hastily it driveth away the fault and the sore from the eyes.

FEVER FUGE, or the lesser Curmel. For sore of eyes, take this same wort's juice; smear the eyes therewith; it heals the thinness of the sight (weakness of vision). Mingle also honey thereto; it benefits similarly dim eyes, so that the brightness (of vision) is restored. If one then fall into this mischief, take a good handful of this same wort, seethe it in wine or in ale, so that of the wine there be an ambur or jug full; have it stand three days; take then every day when there may be occasion, a half sextarius, mix with honey; then let him drink this fasting.

POPPY. For sore of eyes, that is what we denominate blearedness, take the root of this wort, which the Greeks name *mekona*, and the Romans *papaver album*, and the Engle call white poppy, or the stalk, with the fruit, lay it to the eyes.

CELANDINE. For dimness of eyes and soreness and obstruction (*albugo*) take juice of this wort, beaten out of the roots, let that be well pounded with old wine and honey and pepper together, then smear the eyes inwardly. Also, we have found that some men have smeared their eyes with the milk of this same wort, and it was thereby better with them. Again for eyes getting dim, take ooze of this same wort, or the blossoms wrung out, and mixed with honey; mingle then gently hot ashes thereto, and seethe together in a brazen vessel; this is a special leechdom for dimness of eyes.

CHEADLE (*Mercurialis perennis*). For sore of eyes and swelling, take leaves of this same wort, pounded in old wine: lay that to the sore.

HOUNDS HEAD (*Antirrhinum orontium*). For sore of eyes and swelling, take roots of this wort, seethe them in water, and then bathe the eyes with the water; soon it relieves the sore.

RUE. For sore of eyes and swelling, take this same wort rue, well pounded lay it to the sore, also the root pounded, and smear therewith; it well amendeth the sore. For dimness of eyes, the leaves of this same wort, give them (to the patient) to eat fasting, and give (them him) to drink in wine.

RUE (*Ruta Montana*). For dimness of the eyes and for an evil cut, take leaves of this wort, sodden in old wine, then put the extract into a glass vessel; afterwards anoint with the fluid.

BASIL (*Clinopodium vulgare*). For sore and swelling of eyes, pound this same wort in good wine, smear the eyes therewith; thou shalt heal them.

MARCHE (*Apium*). For sore and for swelling of eyes, take this wort, well pounded with bread; lay this to the eyes.

SOUTHERNWOOD (*Artemisia abrotanon*). For sore of eyes, take this same wort, sodden with the wort which is called cydonia, and then pounded with a loaf, as if thou shouldst work a poultice; lay this to the sore, it will be relieved. N.B. this wort is of two kinds, the one is wife, or female, the other wer, or male; and they have in all things alike might against the things of which here before we quoth.

SEMPERVIVUM SEDIFORME. For erysipelatous inflammations, and for sore of eyes, and for foot addle, or gout, take this wort, except the root, pound with smede, or fine flour, in the manner in which thou mightest work up a poultice, lay it to these infirmities; it will alleviate them.

ORPINE, or Livelong. Pounded with meal this wort healeth sore eyes.

ELDER (*Sambucus nigra*). For mickle heat and swelling of the eyes, take the self same wort, mingled with meal, and wrought to a cataplasm; lay to the eyes, they be relieved.

MILOTIS. This wort thou shalt take up in the waning of the moon, in the month which hight August; take then the root of this wort, and bind it to a yarn thread, and hang it to thy neck; that year thou shalt not feel dimness of thine eyes, or if it befall thee, it suddenly shall depart, and thou shalt be hale. This leechcraft is a proved one.

This ends the *Herbarium*. We miss from the descriptions any of the herb eyebright, or euphrasy, also fennel and mallows, which in later times were sovereign cures for ophthalmic conditions. Both the latter herbs find mention in this *Herbarium*, but not in an ophthalmic capacity. We see that the Anglo-Saxon leech relied principally on extracts from the roots or leaves in water, wine or honey. From the frequent mention of the word poultice, we can imagine that the practitioner in those far-off times was much addicted to this old-fashioned and rather septic remedy.

The *Medicina de Quadripedibus* gives the medicinal virtues of the parts of animals, arranged under the headings of the particular animals. As can be imagined all sorts of nastiness find a place, but the eye for the most part is lucky in not having dung or urine advised for its ailments. The following are the ophthalmic portions:

For dimness of eyes, take a foxes gall mingled with honey of dumbledore* (Latin, *cum melle attico*), and applied to the eyes, it healeth.

For sore of eyes, a hares lung set on and bound fast thereto; the sore will be healed. For dimness of eyes, a hares gall mingled with honey, and smeared with, brighteneth the eyes. For sore of eyes, a hares liver sodden is good to drink in wine, and to bathe the eyes with the broth.

For the men who from the tenth hour of the day see not, let them receive with their eyes the smoke of the same drink, and reek them with the broth; and let them wet the liver, and rub and smear therewith.

For brightness of eyes, gall of a wild buck mingled with field bees honey, and smeared on; the brightness cometh to them.

For dimness of eyes, mingle together a wood goats gall and a little of wine; smear therewith thrice; then be they healed.

For heat and pricking of eyes, new goats cheese set upon the eyes with the eyelids; quickly will be amends for him (the man).

To remove away eye pain (*ad glaucomata*, Latin) take a wolfs right eye, and prick it to pieces, and bind it to the suffering eye; it maketh the sore to wane, if it frequently be smeared therewith.

Mingle with field bees honey (*melle attico*), a bulls gall, against obscurity and darkness of the eyes, put it upon the eyes; wonderfully it healeth.

For pain and pricking sensation in the eyes, break to pieces a hounds head; if the right eye ache, take the right eye; if the left ache, take the left eye, and bind it on externally; it healeth well.

Among the fly-leaf leechdoms occur the following which have reference to the eyes:

This is the best eyesalve for eye pain, and for mist, and for pin, and for worms, and for itchings, and for eyes running with teardrops and for every known swelling: take feverfue blossoms, and dills blossoms,

* Dumbledore—a bumble bee.

and thunder clovers blossoms, and hammer worts blossoms, and wormwood of two kinds, and pulegium, and the netherward part of a lily, and coloured dill, and lovage, and pellitory, and pound the worts together, and boil them together in harts marrow or in his grease, and mingle oil besides; put them a good mickle into the eyes, and smear them outwardly and warm at the fire; and this salve helpeth for any swelling, to swallow it and to smear with it, on whatever limb it may be.

This is efficacious for an eyesalve: take yellow stone (ochre), and salt stone (rock salt), and pepper, and weigh them in a balance, and drive them through a cloth, and put of all equally much, and put all together, and drive again through a linen cloth; this is a tried leech-craft.

The following note on beet might give some credence to the view that our Anglo-Saxon forefathers recognised some connection between the eyes and chronic headache:

For old and constant head ache, pound the wort which hight beet, and rub up on the temples and top of the head, thou shalt wonder at the leechdom. Again for the same, pound celandine in vinegar and smear the head therewith above the eyes: the man shall soon be better.

The last ophthalmic leechdom in the first volume is for pain in the eye.

It is, take the netherward part of a bulrush, pound it, and wring it through a hair cloth, and add salt; then squeeze it into the eye.

Bald's leech book begins with a list of the contents; the first two paragraphs may be transcribed here.

Leechdoms against all infirmities of the head, and whence comes ache of all or of the half head (hemicrania) and cleansings and swilling against filth and ratten to the health of the head; and how one must tend a broken head, and how if the brain be out.

Leechdoms against all tenderness of the eyes, against mists of the eyes, either of an old or of a young man, and whence that comes, and against white spot and against tears of eyes, and against speck on eyes, against imminutions (contractions of the pupil) and if a man be bleareyed, against pocks on eyes, and against figs (possibly hordeola) and against worms, or insects; and eye salves of every kind.

The leechdoms for headache are for the most part not worth recording, but the following is of interest:

For head wark, take elecampane and groundsel and fen cress and gitrife, boil them in water, make them steam upon the eyes, when it is hot, and rub about the eyes with the worts so hot.

Bald's leechdoms for the eyes are as follows:

Leechdoms for mistiness of the eyes; take juice or blossoms of celandine, mingle with honey of dumble dores (*melle attico*) introduce it into a brazen vessel, half warm it neatly on warm gledes, till it be sodden. This is a good leechdom for dimness of eyes. For the same mingle the juice of wild rue, dewey and bruised, mingle with equally much of filtered honey, smear the eyes with that. For mistiness of eyes many men, lest their eyes should suffer the disease, look into cold water and then are able to see far; that harmeth not the vision, but much wine drinking and other sweetened drinks and meats, and those especially which remain in the upper region of the wamb and cannot digest, but there form evil humours and thick ones; leek and cole-wort and all that are so austere are to be avoided, and care must be had that a man lie not in bed in day time supine; and cold and wind and reek and dust, these things and the like to these every day are injurious to the eyes. For mistiness of eyes, take green fennel, put it into water for thirty days in a crock (earthen vessel), one that is pitched on the outside, fill it then with rain water; after that throw off the fennel and with the water every day wash the eyes and open them. Again, from the vapour and steam of ill juices and from nausea cometh mist of eyes, and the sharpness and corrupt humour causes that, against which this is to be done. For mist of eyes, take of celandine juice a spoon full, another of fennels, a third of southern-woods juice, and two spoon measures of the tear of honey (virgin honey that drops without pressure), mingle them together and then with a feather put some into the eyes in the morning and when it be midday, and again at evening after that, when it is dried up and spent; for sharpness of the salve, take milk of a woman who hath child, apply it to the eyes.

Again, a noble craft. Take equal quantities of balsam and of virgin honey, mix together and smear with that.

Again, for the same, juice of celandine and sea water; smear and bathe the eyes therewith. It is then most advisable that thou take juice of celandine and of mugwort and of rue, of all equal quantities, add honey to it, and balsam, if thou have it, put it then into such a vessel (probably a covered vessel), that thou may seethe it with glue and make use of it. It does much good.

For mist of eyes, salt burnt and rubbed fine and mixed with dumble dores honey; smear therewith.

Again, juice of fennel and of rose and of rue, and dumble dores honey, and kids gall, mixed together; smear the eyes with this. Again, lay upon the eyes green coriander rubbed fine and mixed with woman milk.

Again, let him take a hares gall and smear with it.

Again, live perriwinkles burnt to ashes; and let him mix the ashes with dumbledores honey.

Again, the fatty parts of all river fishes melted in the sun and mingled with honey; smear with that.

For mist of eyes, juice of betony beaten with its roots and wrung, and juice of yarrow and of celandine, equally much of all, mingle together, apply to the eye. Again, mingle pounded root of fennel with the purest honey, then seethe at a light fire cleverly to the thickness of honey. Then put it in a brazen ampulla, and when need be, smear with it, this driveth away the eye mists, though they be thick.

For mist of eyes again, wring out juice of celandine or of the blossoms of it, and mingle with dumbledores honey, put it in a brazen vessel, then make it lukewarm cleverly on warm gledes, or on ashes, till it be done. That is a unique medicine for dimness of eyes.

Some avail themselves of the juice singly, and anoint the eyes with that. For mist of eyes again; juice of ground ivy and juice of fennel; set equal quantities of both in an ampulla, then dry in the hot sun, and smear the inward part of the eyes with that. For mist of eyes again smear earthgalls juice, that is herdwort, on the eyes, the vision will be by it sharper. It thou addest honey thereto, that is of good effect. Further take a good bundle of the same wort, introduce it into a jug full of wine, and seethe three days in a close vessel; and when it is sodden, wring out the wort, and drink of the ooze sweetened with honey every day, after a nights fasting, a bowl full.

The eyes of an old man are not sharp of sight; than (sic) shall he wake up his eyes with rubbings, with walkings, with ridings, either so that a man bear him or convey him in a wain. And they shall use little and careful meats, and comb their heads and drink wormwood before they take food. Then shall a salve be wrought for unsharp-sighted eyes; take pepper and beat it, and beetle nut and a somewhat of salt and wine; that will be a good salve.

For much eye ache. Many a man hath mickle ache in his eyes. Work him then groundsel and bishopwort (betony) and fennel, boil all the worts in water, milk is better, make that throw up a reek on the eyes. Again, let him mingle with wine celandine and woodbines leaves and the herb cuckoosour (*Oxalis Acetosella*).

Again for much eye ache, pound in wine the nether part of crop-leek (possibly *Allium sativum*) and the nether part of Wihtmars wort (perhaps *Cochlearia anglica*), and let it stand for two days. For pearl, an eye salve; take ashes of broom and a bowl full of hot wine, pour this by a little at a time thrice on the hot ashes, and pour that then into a brass or a copper vessel, add somewhat of honey and mix together, apply to the infirm mans eyes, and again wash the eyes in a clean wyll (spring). For pearl on the eye, apply the gall of a hare, warm, for about two days, it flieth from the eyes. Against white spot, take an unripe sloe, and wring the juice of it through a cloth on the eye, soon, in three days the spot will disappear, if the sloe be green. Against white spot, mingle together vinegar and burnt salt (a substitute for sal ammoniacum) and barley meal, apply it to the eye, hold thine hand a long while on it.

For pearl, an eye salve; take seed of celandine or the root of it, rub it into old wine and into honey, add pepper, let it stand for a night by the fire, use it when thou wilt sleep. Against white spot, boil in butter the nether part of ox-slip (*Primula veris elatior*) and alder (*Alnus glutinosa*) rind.

In case the eyes be tearful, juice of rue, and goats gall and dumble-dores honey, of all equal quantities. If eyes be tearful, add to sweetened wine ashes of harts horn. Work an eye salve for a wen, take cropleek and garlic, of both equal quantities, pound them well together, take wine and bullocks gall, of both equal quantities, mix with the leek, put this then into a brazen vessel, let it stand nine days in the brass vessel, wring out through a cloth and clear it well, put it into a horn, and about night time apply it with a feather to the eye; the best leechdom.

For a wen on the eye, take hollow cress (*Gentiana campestris*), roast it, apply it to the eye, as hot as possible. (N.B. Wisps or styes are still called wuns in Devonshire.)

For eye ache, let him work for himself groundsel and bishopwort and beewort (*Acorus calamus*), and fennel, boil all the worts in water; milk is better.

For ache of eyes, take the red hove (*Glechoma hederacea*), boil it in sour beer or in sour ale, and bathe the eyes in the bath, the oftener the better.

For eye ache, take twigs of withewind (*Convolvulus sepium*), pound them, boil them in butter, apply them to the eyes.

Work an eye salve thus; take nut kernels and wheat grains, rub them together, add wine, strain through a cloth, then apply to the eyes. For acute pain and ache of eyes, mingle well crumbs of white bread and pepper and vinegar, lay this on a cloth, bind it on the eyes for a night. Thus shall a man work an eye salve, take the nether part of strawberry plants and pepper, pound them well, put them on a cloth, bind them fast, lay them in sweetened wine, make somebody drop one drop into the eyes. Work an eye salve thus; leaves of wood-bind (*Convolvulus*), woodmarche (*Apium graveolens*), strawberry plants, southern wormwood (*Artemisia abrotanon*), green hellebore, celandine, pound the worts together much, mingle with wine, put in a copper vessel or keep in a brazen vat, let it stand seven days or more, wring the worts very clean, add pepper, and sweeten very lightly with honey, put subsequently into a horn, and with a feather put one drop into the eyes. Work an eye salve thus: take beetle nut (?) and sulfur, Greek olusatrum (*Smyrnium olustratum*) and burnt salt, and of pepper most, grind all to dust, sift through a cloth, put it on a fawns skin, let him keep it about himself, lest it get moist. Introduce a small quantity into the eyes with a tooth pick; afterwards let him rest himself and sleep, and then wash his eyes with clean water, and let him look in the water, *that is keep his eyes open under water*. Work eye salve thus; pound thoroughly cummin and a strawberry plant, and souse with sweetened wine, put into a copper vessel or into a brazen one, let it stand many nights, wring the wort through a cloth and clear the liquid thoroughly, then apply to the eyes when thou may wish to rest; if the salve be too biting, sweeten it with honey. For imminution of the eyes, take olusatrum, mingle with spittle, anoint the eyes outwardly not inwardly.

For imminutions, the nether part of the herb ashthroat (*Verbena officinalis*), chewed in the mouth and wrung through a cloth, and applied to the eye, wonderfully healeth. In case a man be blear eyed, take agrimony, boil it thoroughly down to the third part, wash the eyes frequently with that. For a pock or pustule in the eyes, take woad and ribwort (*Plantago lanceolata*), and brooklime (*Veronica beccabunga*), boil in milk, in butter is better, and work a fomentation. Boil brooklime and yarrow and wood chervil (*Anthriscus silvestris*) in milk.

For worms (nits) in eyes, take seed of henbane (*Hyoscyamus niger*), shed it on gledes, add two saucers full of water, set them on two sides of the man, and let him sit there over them, jerk the head hither and thither over the fire and the saucers also, then the worms shed themselves into the water. For "dry" disease in the eyes, which is called fig, and in Latin is called churosis (sycosis) the yolk of a hens egg and seed of marche (*Apium*) and olusatrum and garden mint. Again for fig, break to pieces a hock shank unsodden of a sheep, apply the marrow to the eyes. For thick eyelids, take three handfuls of mugwort, three of salt, three of soap, boil them till two parts out of the three of the ooze be boiled away, then preserve in a copper vessel. For him who hath thick eyelids, take a copper vessel, put therein cathartic seeds and salt there among, take celandine and bishopwort and cuckoosour and attorlothe and springwort (*Euforbia lathyris*) and English carrot, and a somewhat of radish, and ravens foot (*Ranunculus ficaria*), then wash them all, then pour wine on; let it stand, strain again into the copper vessel; then let it stand fifteen nights and the dregs will be good. Have with thee clean curds and introduce into the vessel on which the dregs are, as much of the curd as may cleave thereon. Then scrape the scrapings off the vessel, that will be a very good salve for the man who hath thick eyelids.

Bald's formularies for the eye end here. The following are taken from the third of the leech books mentioned above:

For swollen eyes, take a live crab, put his eyes out, and put him alive again into water, and put the eyes upon the neck of the man who hath need; he will soon be well. Work a good eye salve thus; take celandine and bishopwort, wormwood, woodmarche, leaves of woodbind; put equal quantities of all, pound them well, put them into honey, and into wine, and into a brazen vessel, or a copper one; put in of the wine two parts in three, and a third part of the honey, order it so that the liquor may just overrun the worts; let it stand for seven nights, and wrap it up with a piece of stuff; strain the drink through a clean cloth, put it again into that ilk vessel, use as occasion may be.

The man who putteth upon his eyes for about thirty nights, part of the suet of a fox, he will be for ever healthy.

If there be a mist before the eyes, take a childs urine and virgin honey, mingle together of both equal quantities, smear the eyes therewith on the inside.

Again, mingle together a crabs gall, and a salmons, and an eels, and field bees honey, smear the eyes inwardly with the salve.

Against a white spot in the eye; rub to dust burnt salt, and swails apple, and olusatrum, of all equal quantities, rub to dust, and put on the eyes, wash lightly with spring water, smear afterwards with womans milk.

If there are worms in the eyes, scarify the lids within, apply to the scarifications the juice of celandine; the worms will be dead and the eyes healthy. If flesh wax on eyes, wring wormwort into the eyes, till they are well.

If red sponges wax on the eyes, drop on them hot culvers blood, or swallows, or womans milk, till the sponges be got rid of. If the eyes are bleared, take dry rue and virgin honey, mingle together, let it stand for three nights, wring through a linen cloth, and afterwards apply to the eyes. Work a good dry salve for dim vision thus: take swails apple, and burnt salt, and pepper, and olusatrum, and mastich; rub to dust, sift through a cloth, apply by little and little. Again, reduce to dust mastich, and burnt oyster shell, and use as need be; either hath power to remove white spot from the eyes. Work a smooth eyesalve thus; take butter, boil in a pan, skim the foam off, and purify the butter in a dish; put the clear part into a pan; pound celandine and bishopwort, wood marche, boil thoroughly, strain through a cloth; use as need may be.

For imminutions, and for all pain of the eyes; chew wolfscomb, then wring the ooze through a purple cloth upon the eyes, at night, when the man has a mind to rest, and in the morning apply the white of an egg.

The contents of the third volume are of a more varied character than those of the earlier volumes. Various recipes are given, and a good deal of space is devoted to dreams, charms, and a glossary.

There is a good deal of similarity about the recipes, and it seems best to abstract them, rather than to give them in full.

The following eye salves are vaunted. Rub up aloes into vinegar, smear the head therewith, and put it into the eyes. Put into a horn wine and pepper, and into the eyes when you wish to go to bed. Take the nether part of strawberry and pepper, put them into a cloth, lay them in sweetened wine, drop from the cloth a drop into either eye, if eyes are stopped up, take a crabs gall and white mint, wood lettuce and a salmons gall, collect them, drip into the eye through a coloured linen cloth and a little of the ooze of arum, then the eye recovers. The best eye salve is made with dumbledores honey, foxes grease, and a roebucks marrow, mingled together. For pock on the eye, take marrow, soap, and a hinds milk, mix, and whip up, let it stand till it be clear put the clear liquor into the eye; with God's help the pock shall go away. We are next given an all-in policy against eye wark, mist, wen, worms, itch, bleared eyes and all strange swellings. A goodly mixture of worts is boiled with harts marrow or grease, and of the result, a "good much" is put into the eyes and smeared on the outside, warm at the fire. If eyes are bleared, take green rue, pound it small and wash with dumbledores honey or with down honey, wring through a linen cloth on the eye as long as needful. Another recipe for pock in the eye is to take verdigris and a hinds milk, mix and whip up, let it stand till it be clear, then put of the clear stuff into the eye, and with God's help, etc. For an eye salve, take aloes and zedoary, laurel berries and pepper, shave them small, and lay fresh cows butter in water, then take a broad whetstone and rub the butter "on the whetstone with copper so that it may be pretty tough" then add some part of the worts thereto, and put the paste into a brass vessel, let it stand there for nine days and let someone turn it every day; afterwards melt it in the same brass vessel, strain through a cloth, then put it into whatever vessel thou wilt, use it when need be. This is good for all infirmities of the eyes. For sore of eyes sing this Latin prayer "Sana Domine, oculos hominis istius—sicut sanasti oculos Tobiae sancti, et sicut aperuisti oculus duorum cecorum".

For blindness of the eyes. This shall avail for tenderness of the eyes, as Hippocrates the leech made it known, that is to say first that the sore cometh upon the eyes with much heat, as whiles it cometh on with moisture, so that they are swollen, and at whiles without sore-ness, so that they grow blind, and at whiles from the fluxes which run from the eyes. They must then be thus cured. If the disorder cometh from dry heat, then take a cloth and dip it in water, and wash the eyes, then put a cupping horn on the temples; and if they turn blind with-out any soreness, give satureia, savory, to drink, and he will be healed; and eftsoons if any thing fouleth the eyes within, take mead or womans milk, and put it into the eyes.

For bleared eyes; work a poultice like a little cake with pounded leaves of verbena, and lay it on the eyes for a day and a night. Or make a poultice with olusatrum, honey and egg-white, mix and lay to the eyes. New cheese can be used in the same way.

This shall be for dimness of eyes, which the Greeks name glauco-mata. Take three spoons of womans milk, and celandine, one spoon full, and aloes and crocus, (called) saffron in French, and mix, and squeeze through a linen cloth, and then put the salve into the eye.

This shall be for tenderness for eyes, which are sores in the eye roots. Take myrtle berries and lay them in honey, and then take the berries and lay them to the eyes, that the eyes may swell; then take rue and pound it, and mix ashes therewith, and lay them to the eyes, at first it biteth them; swill the eyelids; and after that it cleverly healeth them.

For those who cannot see from sunrise to sunset.

For nyctalopia, that is in our language, those who are able to see nothing after sunrise, till he again go to his setting. This then is the leechcraft which thereto belongeth. Take a knee cap of a buck, and roast it, and when the roast sweats, then take the sweat, and smear therewith the eyes, and after that let the blind eat the same roast; and then take a new asses tord, and squeeze it, and then let him take the ooze, and smear the eyes therewith and it will soon be better with them.

For stye. Take barley meal and knead it with honey, lay it to the eyes: this leechcraft has been tested by many men. Eftsoons, take bean meal and soap, mix, and lay to the eyes.

The dreams contain little of ophthalmic interest. To see oneself blind betokens hindrance. To see onions betokens sore of eyes.

The last nostrum I propose to transcribe is as follows:

This eye salve is good for annoyance of every sort in the eyes, for pin, and for web, for dimness, for wateriness, for insects and for dead flesh. Take a new crock; let it be set in the earth up to the brim, and these worts, minced very small be put into the crock, and on the top of these grout (?) or some liquid, that they may be thoroughly moistened; that is to say, bishopwort of two kinds, and glap, and ribwort and yarrow, and cinqfoil, daisey, and sinfull, and brown hove. After that let a brazen vessel, a dish, or bowl, be scoured in the lower part, till it quite shine; smear all the shining surface lightly with virgin honey. Then put this upon the crock, so that the vapour may strike upwards, then within three days wet thy finger with thy spittle and spatter the dish by little and little. And thence take a good eye salve.

Let virgin honey, and wine, and juice of rue be mixed together, and in equal quantities be put into a copper vessel, or a latten or a brazen one. Thence take a good eye salve.

CHAPTER III

Ophthalmology in the first three centuries after the Norman Conquest

BEFORE the Conquest the records of this kingdom are scanty, and beyond the Anglo-Saxon pharmacopœia alluded to in the last chapter, most of the ophthalmic notices which we obtain are concerned with miraculous cures in cases of blindness, which are of more interest to theologians than to ophthalmic surgeons. A good example of such a miraculous cure is that related by Herman, the Archdeacon. Yates, in his history of Bury Abbey, p. 99, notices this cure of the blindness of Herfastus, Bishop of Elmham, at the hands of Baldwin, Abbot of Bury, and Physician to Edward the Confessor. At this early date the see of what is now Norwich was in a state of flux. Herfastus, the Bishop, was not satisfied with Elmham and in 1070 moved the see to Thetford and shortly afterwards was meditating the appropriation of Bury for his cathedral. He was injured while riding, by being struck by the branch of a tree, and a violent and painful effusion of blood caused immediate blindness. After having been blind for some time the Archdeacon advised him that no collyrium would avail as long as he meditated any injury to Bury Abbey. "Hasten to Abbot Baldwin that his prayers to God and St Edmund may provide an efficacious remedy." This counsel, at first despised, was afterwards followed. Herman undertook the preliminaries and presented a petition to the Abbot at the festival of St Simon and St Jude. "Baldwin granted the request and the blind Herfastus came to Bury, where he was admonished by Baldwin. They went to the church, where, in the presence of the brethren and some of the great men of the realm, the Bishop declared the cause of his misfortunes; recited the injuries he had conceived against this holy place;

confessed himself culpable; condemned, under an anathema, his advisers, and bound himself by a solemn vow to reject such advice in the future. He then advanced with sighs and tears to the foot of the altar; surrendered his pastoral staff; prostrated himself before God and St Edmund; performed his devotions and received absolution from the Abbot. "Then having made trial of the Abbot's medicines and as I saw by the application of cauteries and collyriums, assisted by the prayers of the brethren, in a short time he returned perfectly healed; only a small obscurity remaining in the pupil of one eye as a memorial of his audacity."

Round, in *Feudal England*, has noticed this case and dated it 1076–9. Baldwin was a favourite of the Confessor and the Conqueror continued to regard him with favour. It will be seen that from five to eight years must have elapsed between the injury and the cure; and while it is idle to speculate on the nature of the blindness, I am inclined to attribute it to cataract. Baldwin's collyria may have caused Herfastus to rub his smarting eyes and he may thereby have dislocated his opaque lenses out of the pupillary area, completely in one eye and partially in the other. It is in this way that Sir John Bland Sutton has accounted for Tobit's miraculous restoration of sight recorded in the Apocrypha. Herfastus died about 1085 and Abbot Baldwin in 1098.

I have collected from time to time a number of early references to ophthalmic conditions from various sources, which may, with advantage, be grouped together in this chapter with some account of what I have called judicial blinding; for which a better name would be penal blinding, as there is no evidence of any judicial trial, as we should conceive it, in most of the recorded cases.

An early example of provision for the blind is found in the Domesday survey of Notts., where the following statement occurs: *In Wareshope tenet quidam cecus unam bovatam in elemosina* *de Rege.* This may be translated: "In Warsop* a certain blind man holds one oxgang in alms of the King" (D.B. vol. 1, fol. 293).

Pollock and Maitland in their *History of the English Law,* vol. 1, p. 241, notice this interesting case. They are speaking of the meaning of the word *elemosina* and state that "at first it would express rather the motive of the gift than a mode of tenure that the gift creates. In Domesday Book it is used in various senses and contexts. In some cases a gift has been made by the King *in elemosina,* but the donee is to all appearances a layman; in one case he is blind, in another maimed; he holds by way of charity, and perhaps his tenure is precarious". Medical references are very rare in Domesday Book and this reference to a blind person is, I believe, unique.

Although blinding as a penalty was in force before the Conquest, as is proved by the deplorable treatment of the brother of Edward the Confessor, the Conqueror was, I think, the first to regularise penal blinding. Among the statutes of the Conqueror, given by Stubbs in *Select Charters,* occurs the following: *Interdicto etiam ne quis occidatur aut suspendatur pro aliqua culpa, sed eruantur oculi, et testiculi abscidantur.* This means that convicted persons were not to be hung or killed, but, instead, to have their eyes destroyed and to be castrated.

Apparently England was in such good order under the iron rule of the Conqueror that the extreme penalty was unnecessary; and we read that a man might go anywhere without fear: "No man durst slay other man, had he never so mickle evil done to the other" (*Chron. Petrib.* 1087).

The blinding of the Confessor's brother referred to above occurred in 1036. The Norman version of this affair is given in Freeman's *Norman Conquest,* vol. 1, pp. 546–7: "After the expedition of Edward (later the Confessor) his younger brother, Alfred, set sail from Wissant, and landed at Dover. As he went onwards

---

* Near Mansfield.

into the country, Godwin met him, received him friendly, and seemingly did homage to him. The Earl and the Aetheling supped together and talked over their plans. But in the night Godwin seized Alfred, tied his hands behind his back, and thus sent him and some of his companions to London to King Harold (Hardicanute). Others he put in prison, others he embowelled. Among those who were sent to London, Harold beheaded Alfred's chief companions, and blinded the Aetheling himself. In that state he was sent to Ely, naked and with his legs tied under his horse's belly. He had not been long at Ely when he died, as the weapon with which his eyes had been cut out had wounded the brain. *Cui dum oculi effoderentur cultro cerebrum violavit mucro*".

Under Henry the First penal blinding seems to have reached its acme, and I doubt if it were much in use after the date of Glanville (A.D. 1180).

Matthew of Westminster, quoted in Holinshed's *Chronicles*, gives the story of the penal blinding of Robert, Duke of Normandy, the Conqueror's eldest son and Henry's elder brother.

The Duke was captured in 1107 and confined at Cardiff. He attempted his escape but was recaptured. "His keepers kept him in close prison advertising the King of his demeanour: whereupon he commanded that the sight of his eies should be put out, but so, as the balles of them should remain unbroken, for the avoiding of a noisome deformitie that would otherwise ensue, if the glassie tunicles should take hurt." The eyes of the unfortunate Duke were probably "stung" out with a red hot needle, much as decoy birds are said to have been treated. This early appreciation of the hideous deformity caused by a double excision does more credit to Henry's powers of observation than to his benevolence.

William of Malmesbury (lib. 4) gives us, in describing the personal appearance of William Rufus, the fact that he had heterochromia iridis; while Matthew Paris, performing a like office for Henry the Third, tells us that the upper lid of one of his eyes hung down so as partially to obscure the eyeball: obviously a case of partial ptosis.

With the settlement of the kingdom after the anarchy of Stephen's reign we find law and order becoming more fixed. Such actions as are recorded in the public records are mainly those in connexion with the devise of landed property, but occasionally we meet with an action for personal injury. This occurs on the Lincolnshire Assize Roll for 1202, which has been edited for the Lincoln Record Society by Mrs Stenton. A certain man appealed another that he had assaulted him in the King's peace and thrust out his eye, so that his sight was maimed in that eye. This was denied by the aggressor, and a trial by ordeal was ordered, but the result of the case is not recorded.

An early example of eyestrain is given by Coulton in his *Social Life in Britain from the Conquest to the Reformation*, as an excerpt from Trevisa's *Higden*, vol. VIII, p. 27, which deals with the model student. "In his childhood he lernede his gramere and was so disesed with the heedache that he hadde non hope to spede afterwards in lore. His moder spak to hym and seide, 'Sone, I trowe that the lewednesse and unsemeliche tonsure that thou useth is the cause of thy woo'; thanne afterwards he usede tonsure as a clark and was hool of al that woo." The weight of the hair as a possible cause for headache is worth remembering, and I myself recollect being told by a female patient, some few years ago, that she had always suffered from headache until her hair was shingled; since that time her headache had practically disappeared.

From the same source (*i.e.* Coulton) we learn of an early case of vanity in the refusal to wear glasses, in a male person: Hoccleve, in the English version of *De Regimine Principum*, 1411–12, says that he had been twenty-four years come Easter in the Privy Seal Office. He groans over his copying, but was too vain to wear glasses.

> Thow foul book, un-to my Lord seye also,
> That pryde ys un-to me so greet a fo,
> That the spectacle forebideth he me,

And hath y-doon of tyme yore ago;
And, for my sighte blyve hastith me fro.
And lackith that that sholde his comfort be,
No wonder thogh thow have no beautee.
Out up-on pryde, causer of my wo
My sighte is hurt thrgh hir adversitee.

I have already alluded to the fact that miraculous restoration of sight is of frequent occurrence in records of the Church from the time of Bede onwards; and two such miracles are recorded by Canon Bannister, in his history of Hereford Cathedral, as occurring at the shrine of St Thomas de Cantilupe, and may be abstracted here. In the bull of canonisation of St Thomas, Pope John the Twenty-Second affirms that accounts of seventeen miracles were thoroughly investigated and proved by faithful testimony. Two of these miracles occurred in cases of blindness; the first in a well-to-do female, who had no obvious reason for making money out of her infirmity. She was stated to have in her blind eyes neither wound, apostheme, tumour, macula, or sickness or any apparent lesion. One must suppose that this was a case either of acute retrobulbar neuritis of a fulminating nature or of hysterical blindness. The other case concerned two small boys, brothers, who obviously were afflicted with catarrhal conjunctivitis. *Mali humores effluebant ex oculis, et aliquando claudebantur palpebrae dictorum oculorum; tunc ipsi oculi inflabantur et putredine congregata in eis denuo palpebrae aperiebantur.*

The belief in springs and wells with miraculous powers of curing sore eyes has probably existed from the earliest times. They may have owed their efficacy partly to the general cleansing effects of the water, partly to salts dissolved in the water, and perhaps chiefly to the psychological effect. The same remarks apply to the belief that rain-water caught on Ascension Day is a highly efficient eye lotion. In a remote parish in North Worcestershire this belief was maintained among the rustics until quite recent times, and may possibly still exist for aught I know to the contrary.

CHAPTER IV

The Founders of British Optics

A GREAT FRANCISCAN TRIAD

I T is generally considered at the present time that the use of spectacles is of comparatively recent development. No specimen prior to the date A.D. 1500 has been preserved; though glasses are occasionally mentioned in old wills from the year 1372 onwards. Greeff asserts that China was not, as has been conjectured, the birthplace of eyeglasses. The story of Nero's emerald is well known; it is usually thought that he used it as an anti-glare glass. On the other hand Wilfrid's beryl seems to have been used, in reading, for its magnifying properties, and as Wilfrid was an English bishop we may credit our country with a very early use of such aids to vision. The Romans were resigned to having their manuscripts read out to them after they had reached the age of fifty years. Ptolemy, in the second century A.D., established the beginnings of optics, and his work was amplified by Al-Hazen (A.D. 996–1038).

Roger Bacon, whose life spanned the greater part of the thirteenth century, is looked upon as the father of British optics; and his fellow Franciscan, John de Peckham, later Archbishop of Canterbury, is credited with the first description of concave glasses and with writing the *Perspectiva Communis*, which became the recognised textbook on optics in Britain. But, besides these two celebrated friars, I wish to advance the view that Roger Bacon's great teacher, Grosseteste, who later in life became Bishop of Lincoln, must be considered worthy of mention in any chapter which deals with the foundation of optics in this country.

Roger Bacon makes frequent mention of Grosseteste and always speaks of him with respect. Stevenson, in his life of Grosseteste (1899), says: "Roger Bacon's estimate of Grosseteste's achievements in the domain of science derives especial value not only from the range of the writer's own attainments but also from the fact that he was not inclined, as a general rule, to praise either his immediate predecessors or his contemporaries. It is well, therefore, to compare and to contrast that estimate with the opinion he formed and repeatedly expressed with regard to the three most widely read writers of his own age, Alexander de Hales, Albertus Magnus and Thomas Aquinas. Of Alexander, the *Doctor Irrefragibilis* of the Franciscans, whose *Summa* was on one occasion proclaimed by an assembly of seventy doctors to be infallible, Bacon declares that the *Summa* in question, though it was as heavy as the weight of a horse, was full of errors, and displayed ignorance of physics, of metaphysics and even of logic. Of Albertus Magnus, the *Doctor Universalis* of the Dominicans, he writes that what is useful in his works might be summed up in a treatise twenty times as short as they are. Thirdly, in speaking of Thomas Aquinas, who, it is true, had not attained at the time Bacon wrote to the commanding position of authority which was afterwards accorded to him in the schools, he couples him with Albertus Magnus, and says that they both became teachers before they had been adequately taught, and lectured on a philosophy and a theology which they had imperfectly learned".

Now Bacon says of Grosseteste in his *Compendium Studii*: "The Lord Robert neglected altogether the books of Aristotle and their methods, and by his own experiments and with the aid of other authors, and by means of other sciences, employed himself in the scientific questions which Aristotle had treated; and he knew and described the questions with which the books of Aristotle deal a hundred thousand times better than they can be understood from the perverse translations of that author". This doubtless refers to Grosseteste's numerous treatises on scientific subjects, such as those on meteorology, on comets, on light, colour, optics and above all to his *Compendium Scientiae*. The importance of these works consisted not only in the additions which he made to existing stocks of knowledge, but in the fact that he gave to experiment the same place in scientific methods which it holds in Bacon's own writings, which lapsed after Bacon's time into disuse for several centuries.

Bacon says in another place: "One man alone had really known the sciences, namely Robert, Bishop of Lincoln, and that while Boethius was the only translator who had an adequate knowledge of languages, the Lord Robert alone, on account of his long life and the wonderful methods which he employed, excelled all men in his knowledge of the sciences". In his work on Mathematics, Bacon says: "Nobody can attain to proficiency in that science by the method hitherto known, unless he devotes to its study thirty or forty years, as is evident from the case of those who have flourished in those departments of knowledge, such as the Lord Robert of holy memory, sometime Bishop of Lincoln, and Friar Adam Marsh, and Master John Hendover, and the like, and that is the reason why so few study that science". And in the *Opus Majus* he writes: "There were found some famous men, such as Robert, Bishop of Lincoln, and Adam Marsh, and several others, who were aware that the power of mathematics is capable of unfolding the causes of all things, and of giving a sufficient explanation of human and divine phenomena; and the assurance of this fact is to be found in the writings of those great men, as, for instance, in their works on the impressions, on the rainbow and the comets, on the generation of heat, on the investigation of geography, on the sphere, and on other questions appertaining both to theology and to natural philosophy". Again: "Few have attained to consummate wisdom in the perfection of philosophy: Solomon attained to it and Aristotle in relation to his times, and in a later age Avicenna, and in our own days the recently deceased Robert, Bishop of Lincoln, and Adam Marsh". Lastly: "Grosseteste knew mathematics and perspective, and there was nothing which he was unable to know; and at the same time he was sufficiently acquainted with languages to be able to understand the saints and philosophers and the wise men of antiquity; but his knowledge of languages was not such as to enable him to effect translations until the latter portion of his life, when he summoned Greeks and caused books on Greek grammar to be brought together from Greece and other countries". Such is a brief account of what Bacon thought of his great master.

ROBERT GROSSETESTE

Robert Grosseteste was born about the year 1175, at Stradbroke, in Suffolk, of humble parentage. Giraldus Cambrensis, in a letter introducing Grosseteste to William de Vere, Bishop of Hereford, calls him *Magister*. The latest possible date for this letter is 1199, for in that year William de Vere died, and from this title of *Magister* it is concluded that when the letter was written, Grosseteste was a regent in arts and at least twenty-four years of age. He may have received his preliminary education at one of the East Anglian monasteries, either Bury, Eye, or Hoxne, and his studies were completed at Oxford and possibly at Paris. At Oxford he certainly learnt law and medicine. As time went by he received ecclesiastical preferment; Pegge makes him a Canon of Chester in 1210. The Salisbury Registers prove him to have been Archdeacon of Wilts. in 1214 and 1220; while in 1224 he was appointed the first Rector of Franciscans at Oxford, by Agnellus de Pisa, Provincial Minister of the Order in England. He was probably, as Archdeacon, transferred from Salisbury to Northampton in 1221. He next exchanged to the archdeaconry of Leicester, which he held till 1231, at which time he resigned all his appointments, save a prebend stall, on account of ill-health. After this he was for a few years at Oxford, and it is probable that his mathematical treatises and his ponderous *Dicta* were composed at this time.

In 1235 he was elected Bishop of Lincoln; thenceforward he is the man of affairs with no time for writing scientific treatises. He was a most efficient bishop and ruled the enormous see of Lincoln, which then and for years afterwards reached from the Humber to the Thames, as it had never been ruled before. In 1245 he had to pay a visit to the Pope at Lyons about a prolonged quarrel which he had with the Dean and Chapter of his see; this was settled in his favour. In the following year he obtained a papal bull to prevent any scholar of Oxford graduating in arts without having passed the usual examinations, *secundum morem Parisiensem*, and without the approval of the Bishop or his nominee. In 1253 occurred the transaction which has done more to make his name respected and popular than any other in his long and active life. Pope Innocent the Fourth ordered Grosseteste to induct Frederick di Lavagna, the Pope's nephew, to a rich canonry at Lincoln, "notwithstanding any exemption or privilege of the church of Lincoln". Grosseteste utterly refused to obey the papal command and Higden, in his *Polychronicon*, calls his letter in answer to the Pope "a sharpe pistle".

Early in October 1253 Grosseteste fell ill at his country seat of Buckden and he died on October the ninth. He was buried in the cathedral church of Lincoln. His death produced the usual crop of portents and we find, later in the century, Peckham writing to friends at Rome, and referring to the power of Grosseteste to raise spirits. Attempts to obtain formal canonisation failed; his "sharpe pistle" was probably too much for the Pope, but he was often spoken of in after days as St Robert. Eighteenth-century antiquaries ascribed the authorship of *De Oculo Morali* to him; this work is now regarded as being by John de Peckham. That late in the seventeenth century he was reckoned one of the most learned men of all time is evidenced by the couplet in *Hudibras*, part 2, canto 3:

> Yet none a greater knowledge boasted,
> Since old Hog Bacon and Bob Grosted.

ROGER BACON, *c.* 1214–1294

It is usually held that Bacon was born at Ilchester in Somerset, although the neighbourhoods of Witney, Oxon. and Bisley, Glos. also have claims to be considered. It would appear that he was well connected and that his family was a wealthy one. In this respect I may state that in an earlier generation a Roger Bacon appears from well-authenticated documents to have been brother to Philip de Columbiéres, whose ancestor, William de Colum-biéres, was one of the Conqueror's companions at Hastings.

Always studious, Bacon in 1267 could write that it was forty years since he first learned the alphabet, and "except for two of those years I have always been *in studio*". He was at Oxford in 1233, when Edmund Riche, who later became Archbishop of Canterbury, "lectured at Oxford in my time". He left Oxford for Paris about 1245, where he heard William of Auvergne, who died in 1248, dispute before the whole University. Bacon is supposed to have returned to Oxford about 1250 and was lecturing there soon afterwards. In or about 1256 he was exiled from England and kept under supervision at Paris for ten years. In 1263 he wrote his *Computus Naturalium*, which attracted the notice of the Cardinal Bishop of Sabina, who, in 1265, became Pope Clement the Fourth. The Pope wrote to Bacon requesting him to send him a fair copy of his works. In this way were born the *Opus Majus*, the *Opus Minus* and the *Opus Tertium*; and, in-credible as it may seem, these three books were written and sent to the Pope in eighteen months. Clement's more liberal views allowed Roger Bacon to return to England at about this time. He was at work on a manual which was to embrace the whole range of sciences as then understood, in the year 1271. His verbal attacks on all classes, including his own order, became more and more violent, and in 1277 and 1278 synods were held at Paris and Oxford to condemn erroneous doctrines. The repres-sive movement extended to the Franciscans and in 1278 Jerome of Arcoli, the Minister General, who later became Pope Nicholas the Fourth, held a chapter at Paris and, among other friars, Roger was condemned, *propter quasdam novitates*. He is believed to have been kept in prison for fourteen years. It is probable that he was released in 1292, in which year was written his *Compendium Studii Theologiae*. He is supposed to have died in 1294, and John Rous says that he was buried at Oxford.

I have dealt superficially with the scientific works of Roger
Bacon in a paper in the *British Journal of Ophthalmology*, January
1928. From this paper I reprint the section dealing with Bacon's
knowledge of optics, which I owed to the kindness of Dr Charles
Singer, who gave me permission to transcribe his chapter on the
invention of the first optical apparatus in vol. II of his *Studies in
the History and Method of Science* (1921). I wish again to acknow-
ledge my indebtedness to Dr Singer for permission to use his
material once more.

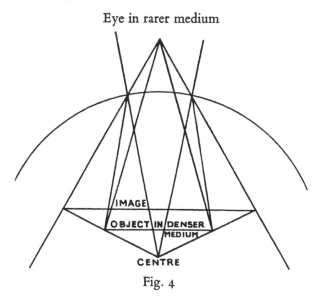

Fig. 4

"The following passages will serve to indicate the stage he had
reached in optical knowledge. It will be observed that in the first of
the passages Bacon figures and refers to the *object* as though it were
itself in the denser medium of which the lens is composed. He thus
confuses the optical action of the lens with that of a liquid in which an
object is immersed. Perhaps he is led to do this by his knowledge
that the optical results of immersion in a liquid had been investigated
by his predecessors, or perhaps by their descriptions of the process of
vision as taking place within the supposed central crystalline sphere
of the eye. It is also apparent that he does not realise the refractive
action of the *plane* surface of his plano-convex lenses.

If anyone examine letters or other minute objects through the medium of crystal or glass or other transparent substance, if it be shaped like the lesser segment of a sphere, with the convex side towards the eye, and the eye being in the air, he will see the letters far better, and they will seem larger to him. For according to our canon (Fig. 4) concerning a spherical medium beneath which the object is placed, the centre being beyond the object, the convexity being towards the eye, all causes agree to increase the size, for the angle in which it is seen is greater, the image is greater, and the position of the image is nearer, because the object is between the eye and the centre. *For this reason such an instrument is useful to old persons and to those with*

Eye in rarer medium

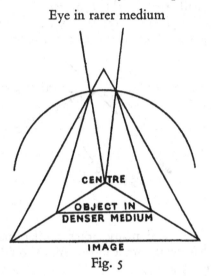

Fig. 5

weak eyes, for they can see any letter, however small, if magnified enough. But if a larger segment of a sphere be employed, then, according to our canon (Fig. 5) the size of the angle is increased, and also the size of the image, but propinquity is lost because the position of the image is beyond the object, the reason being that the centre of the sphere is between the eye and the object seen. Therefore such an instrument is not of so much use as the smaller portion of a sphere.

Objects are greater when the vision is refracted; for it easily appears by the above-mentioned canons that very large objects may seem to be very small and conversely, and those at a great distance away may seem very near and conversely. For we can so form glasses and so arrange them with regard to our sight and to objects that the rays are refracted and deflected to any place we wish, so that we see the object near at hand or far away beneath whatever angle we desire. And so we can read the smallest letters or count grains of sand or dust from an incredible distance owing to the magnitude of the angle beneath which we see them, and again the largest objects close at hand might be scarcely visible owing to the smallness of the angle beneath which we view them; for *it is on the size of the angle on which this kind of vision depends, and it is independent of distance save per accidens.* So a boy can appear a giant, a man seem a mountain, and in any size of angle whatever, for we can see a man under as large an angle as though he were a mountain and make him appear as near as we desire. So a small army might seem very large, and though far away appear near, and conversely: *so, too, we could make sun, moon, and stars apparently descend here below,* and similarly appear above the

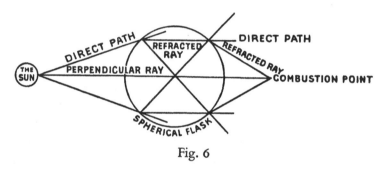

Fig. 6

heads of our enemies, and many other similar marvels could be brought to pass, that the ignorant mortal mind could not endure the truth. (*Opus Majus,* part 5.)

As to double refraction, what is causally manifest with regard to it we can verify in many ways by the results of experiment. For if anyone holds a crystal ball or a round urinal flask filled with water in the strong rays of the sun, standing by a window in face of the rays, he will find a point in the air between himself and the flask at which point, if any easily combustible substance is placed, it will catch fire and burn, which would be impossible unless we suppose a double refraction. For a ray of the sun coming from a point in the sun through the centre of the flask is not refracted, because it falls perpendicularly on flask, water, and air passing through the centre of each (Fig. 6)....But all the other rays given forth at the same point in the sun from which this perpendicular ray comes are necessarily refracted in the body of the flask, because they fall at oblique angles, and since the flask is denser than air, the refraction passes between the straight path and the perpendicular drawn from the point of refraction to the centre of the flask. And when it passes out again into the air, then, since it comes upon a less dense body, the straight path passes between the refraction and the perpendicular drawn from the point of refraction, so that the refracted ray may fall upon the first perpendicular which comes without refraction from the sun. *Now since an infinite number of rays are given off from the same point of the sun, and one only falls perpendicularly on the flask, all the others are refracted and meet at one point on the perpendicular ray which is given off along with them from the sun, and this point is the point of combustion.* On it are collected an infinite number of rays, and the concentration of light causes combustion. But this concentration would not take place except by double refraction, as shown in the diagram. (*Opus Majus,* part 7.)

Glasses (perspicua) can be so constructed that objects at a very great distance appear to be quite close at hand, and conversely. Thus we read the smallest letters from an incredible distance, number objects however small, and make the stars appear as near as we wish.... Also objects can be made to appear so that the greatest seems the least, and conversely; what are high appear low and short, and conversely; and what is hidden appears manifest.... But among the more subtle powers of construction is this of directing and concentrating rays by means of (instruments of) different forms and reflections at any distance we wish, where whatever is subjected to them is burned.... But greater than any such design or purpose is that the heavens might be portrayed in all their length and breadth on a corporeal figure moving with their diurnal motion, and this would be worth a whole kingdom to a wise man. Let this, then, be sufficient as an example, although an infinite number of other marvels could be set forth. (*De Secretis Operibus Artis et Naturae.*)"

Dr Singer states in a footnote that the above passages are translated from Dr J. H. Bridges's *The Opus Majus of Roger Bacon,* Oxford, 1897, and J. S. Brewer's *Fratris Rogeri Baconi opera quaedam hactenus inedita,* London, 1859.

It must be confessed, I fear, that Roger's contemporaries found him "gey ill to live wi'"; but it is a pleasing thought that in spite of hardship, neglect and obloquy, he refused to be muzzled, and that he continued to the end of his life writing, ever writing and thinking about three centuries ahead of his time; and I, for one, shall always consider him a far greater man, considering the age in which he lived, than his namesake, Francis, Baron Verulam and Viscount St Albans. Roger's views may have been too much for the ecclesiastics of his age, but he did not have to confess that he had been guilty of corrupt practices.

JOHN DE PECKHAM

A memoir of John de Peckham was contributed to the *British Journal of Ophthalmology* in February 1929 by Miss Ida Mann and myself. I have drawn on this for much of what follows. Peckham, like Grosseteste, was of humble parentage. The date of his birth is not known, nor is his birthplace ascertained with certainty. It was in one of the southern counties, Sussex, Surrey, or Kent, and possibly occurred at Chichester. He was educated at Lewes Priory and Oxford. Later on he went to Paris and took the degree of S.T.P., corresponding to the modern D.D. At about this time he joined the Franciscan Order, and ever afterwards, even when Archbishop of Canterbury, called himself *Frater Johannes*. In 1277 he was appointed Provincial Minister of the Franciscans in England, and thenceforward he appears as a statesman and man of affairs. He found it necessary to go to Rome to study Canon Law and by his ability attracted the notice of the Pope, who appointed him *Causarum Auditor* and *Lector Palatii*; on receiving this post he resigned his office in England and was at Rome for two years. He was still there when the Archbishop of Canterbury, Kilwardby, arrived to take his place in the *Curia* as a Cardinal. The latter died at Rome and the Pope appointed Peckham to the vacant archbishopric, and he, "sore against his inclination", was consecrated by the Pope on February 10th, 1279. The Chapter at Canterbury had previously chosen Robert Burnell, Chancellor of England and Bishop of Bath and Wells, to succeed Kilwardby; and how it was that Edward the First allowed the Pope to nominate and consecrate

Peckham does not appear. It is probable that the Pope was within his rights, because, according to Canon Law, if a bishop died in *curia*, the appointment of a successor belonged of right to the Pope, and it is probable that both Edward and Burnell thought of Peckham as a theologian rather than as a man of affairs and, in the unsettled state of the Scottish border and Welsh March, preferred to have a churchman at Canterbury as less likely to interfere with their plans.

Peckham's Register is at Lambeth and, printed in the Rolls Series, forms three bulky octavo volumes. He was a strict disciplinarian and stern in correcting abuses; Edward the First made use of him as an ambassador to the Welsh on more than one occasion. Peckham died, according to Hook in his *Lives of the Archbishops of Canterbury*, on December 8th, 1294. He is buried in the Martyrdom in the cathedral. Peckham was a prolific author; his books are mainly on theology and science and he was the author of a few poems of a religious character.

Trice Martin, in his introduction to Peckham's Register, vol. III, gives a list of his works which fills more than two pages. He notices the scientific works first of all, beginning with the *Perspectiva Communis*, published at Milan in 1482. He notes that the book is concerned with the elementary propositions of optics, "such as the incidence of rays of light, reflection and refraction, the non-existence of colour without light, the construction of the eye, the appearance of objects at a distance (viz. spheres as planes and squares as oblongs); and spherical, cylindrical and concave mirrors, whose property of conveying heat is described". The work is divided into three parts, of which in later editions the first two are thus entitled, *De iis quae objiciuntur visu*; *De radiorum visibilium reflexione et eorundem effectibus*. The third part treats of the stars, the rainbow and the milky way. The Venice edition, by J. Baptist Sessa (1504), contains some new figures. It is dedicated to Paulo Trivisano, a Venetian noble. The Leipzig edition contains an odd variation on the author's name in the title, which reads *Perspectiva Johannis Pisani Anglici etc.* Peckham's description of concave refracting surfaces is famous as being the first mention of this section of optics. According to Hirschberg (*Geschichte der Augenheilk. in Europ. Mittelalter*), Pope Leo the Tenth, in 1475, was painted by Raphael, wearing concave glasses. There are two copies in MS. of his *Theorica Planetarum* in the British Museum, both dating from the middle of the fifteenth century. In Arundel MS. 83, fol. 123 *b*, there is an illumination of the *Sphera Secundum fratrem J. de Peckham, archiepiscopum*, executed not long after the Archbishop's death. It is an astronomical work. As stated earlier in this chapter, Peckham is now credited with the authorship of the *De Oculo Morali*. This book is a queer medley of saintly saws and religious dogmas; it is obviously founded on the *Perspectiva Communis*, as many of the propositions in it are those which are found in the former book. I believe that the same odd hash of the Archbishop's name is found in those editions which have a title-page; and it is of course possible that Grosseteste, who must have been acquainted with the optics of Al-Hazen, may have been the author of the *De Oculo Morali*. I contributed a short note on the authorship of this book to the *British Journal of Ophthalmology* in the year 1931.

PLATE II

British Museum. Sloane MS. 75, fol. 146

JOHN OF ARDERNE'S *DE CURA OCULORUM*

CHAPTER V

Ophthalmology from A.D. 1300 to A.D. 1600

FROM the end of the thirteenth to that of the fifteenth century there is a blank in ophthalmological history, broken only, so far as I know, by the small tract *De Cura Oculorum* of John of Arderne. Sir D'Arcy Power included a short account of this booklet among the lesser writings of Arderne, in a paper read at the XVIIth International Congress of Medicine held in London in August 1913. He would appear to have used both the Latin text as well as an early English translation of it. He states that it lacks originality and is rather laboured, much of it being taken from Lanfranc. It certainly does not contain any of those personal touches which make the surgical writings of John of Arderne of such vivid interest. In fact the most interesting and at the same time valuable part of the tract is in the sentence, sandwiched in towards the end, where, after extolling the good effects of human urine as an eye wash, he says: "Know all men present and to come that I Master John of Ardern and the least of surgeons wrote this little book with my own hand at London in the first year of the reign of King Richard the Second and at my age of seventy years". The year in question is 1377, and so John of Arderne is proved to have been born in or about the year 1307. The page containing this entry is reproduced here.

Mr Harvey Bloom, who copied the manuscript for me, is of the opinion that the manuscript in the British Museum is a copy of Arderne's original script; he thinks that its date is about fifty years later than that mentioned.

I have thought it best to give a fairly full abstract of the contents of this tract and to print the Latin text in an appendix. I have been much helped by Mr Harvey Bloom in the translation of it; but in one or two places the meaning is not clear and I have decided to give a very free rendering of the sense.

A collyrium for sick eyes, whether it shall be from injury or from a flux of humours, can be made with the white of a raw egg well beaten up to which is added a half-part of rose-water and then woman's milk, to which is added the weight of a penny or a halfpenny of crocus which is to be dissolved in the aforesaid liquor: two or three drops of the solution are to be placed in the eye.

An *emplastrum* (which seems to mean a poultice) may be made of fine shreds of linen soaked in the aforesaid liquor in which the crocus has been placed and placed immediately over the eye. This provides much aid, it mitigates pain, purifies the blood and softens dryness. The white of an egg soothes immediately, which is pleasant above all else. It constrains the humours lest they run to the eyes and guards the natural humours against dissolution. It purifies and permits no excess of other humours nor spume to come to the eyes and keeps them healthy. The white of an egg which clarifies the eye is of the same quality as the eye. Crocus relieves the redness of the eyes and stays the flux of humours to the eye, it deletes pannus, which is macula of the eye, for it becomes dissolved and wasted away. Rose-water takes away the natural heat in the eye, reprieves the brain which it comforts, increases the natural spirits and has many other conveniences. With this medicine many lesions, however horrible such may be, can be cured; indeed, it was a cure for a certain man whose eye, smitten with a sword, hung down upon his cheek to the size of an egg, who afterwards saw well enough with that same eye. When the aforesaid poultice shall become dry let it be replaced in the aforesaid liquor and when softened applied to the eye. Further, if the eye shall be very much inflamed, the juice of burdock poured in, that is of agrimony, beaten up with white of egg and applied with shreds of linen, it will be well healed for certain. The same juice is made of leaves of elder prepared by me as is said of agrimony; this I have often proved and if to the aforesaid crocus be added it will be the more efficacious.

SWELLING AND DISCHARGE OF THE LIDS OR EYES A CAUSE OF MELANCHOLY

This poultice may be applied, the patient having been first purged with the pills without which I would not like to be: take a sour apple and having cooked it in the cinders, let the rind be removed as is ordered: the white of one egg is added to four apples and a leaf

pounded up, and of this apply with shreds of linen twice daily to the
closed eye. This poultice firstly reduces the swelling of the eye,
secondly collects it into its proper place, thirdly assuages pain and has
recovered the sight according to Lanfranc. And be it known that if
the patient be young much is open to him by phlebotomy from the
vein in the middle of the forehead, the poultice to be applied to the
eyes before he be purged. This removes redness of the eyes and discharge of the lids. The collyrium of brambles which may be of that
bramble that is called *Redebrerecropys* well ground in salt and digested
in white wine to a half of the whole and warmed can be kept for use:
moreover the frontal vein needs this care. Again, aloes epatica
digested in white wine and instilled into the eyes when they are red
is the best remedy. It heals ulceration of the lids, begets good flesh
and corrodes bad flesh. But let the "Licurigum" be powdered and
that minutely, to which is added two parts of oil of roses and one
part of vinegar, being careful that the mixture be gradual and the
result should be a white ointment. This is good for old hot ulcers in
eyes resulting from injury.

Let the yolk of a raw egg be applied with oil of roses to mitigate
the pain. It cures lippitudo. A decoction of roses and galls in rain-
water can be used warm and relieves smarting of the eyes.

Tutty is astringent and is useful in ulcers of the eyes; it keeps the
eyes healthy if it be placed in the underneath part of the eyes.
Further, tutty, nine times heated strongly and then five times
quenched in the urine of a chaste virgin, and four times in rose-
water or white wine, but in the last combustion not quenched in any
solvent but allowed to cool by itself, should afterwards be ground
very fine upon a mill stone and rubbed though a very fine cloth.
Then let it be dissolved in the same liquor in which it was quenched
to a fairly thick solution, which being done the tutty, thus tempered,
is placed in a brass pot well cleaned and (?) scoured and smeared on
the sides and bottom so that it does not run down: afterwards let
there be taken good aloes epatica, powdered not too small and placed
upon slow glowing coals; which done, let the pot be straightway
turned bottom upwards upon the coals so that it may be able to
receive the aloes as it ascends, and thus let a penny be cast into the pot.
It will be dried. After it has been scraped from the pot and dried in
the sun, let it be powdered and again ground up and kept for use;
i.e. the dust. This, thus prepared, deletes macula of the eyes, cools the
burning redness of the eyes and astringes the tears, which comforts
and protects the sight: or a part of the powder and a little lard of a

capon is a useful ointment if first softened and placed in the eye. Or a few drops of the solution of tutty prepared as mentioned by being burnt, powdered and placed in a fine linen cloth and soaked in urine, can be placed when cool in the eye by means of a feather. This helps redness and watering of the eye and clears the sight. Tutty, by itself alone, prepared by the said method or powdered and mixed with keffetine sugar, placed in the lower part of the eye gently eats away pannus and macula while the light of the eye is cleared. It reduces swollen lids, deletes redness of the eye and discharge from the lids, dries the tears and increases the vision, which it strengthens and pre-serves: and this I have proved. These be soothing to the eyes: the milk of a woman warm and freshly placed, the milk of a she-ass, white of egg and the blood of a dove drawn from under the wing. Tutty is found for sale among the apothecaries, a pound of which is sold for twelve or sixteen pence; very fine laminae should be chosen. It is brought from overseas.

According to John of Damascus in all ocular pain and for visual defect one must first consider whether it be from a hot or a cold cause. Let pearls be digested in an acid syrup three or four days: take the digested pearls for a clyster. A morning draught of decoction of mallows evacuates the body. An electuary of juice of roses acidulated with ... twice or thrice renders it more secure; it is to be used with local remedies as may seem expedient to you.

But indeed first let it be digested in cold water mixed with diuretic oxymelle or squills. Let half a clyster be given in the morning. The body is vexed with one ounce of "Ierapige" of Galen (almost certainly holy bitters, *hiera picra*), which can be found at the apothecaries; after proceed with local remedies. The milk of a woman or of an ass with yolk of a raw egg, crocus and oil of roses placed over the eye sufficiently soothes it and disperses the burning of the eyes; it corrects the inflammation and if the juice of wild celery, that is *smallache* (smallage) or vervaine, or portulaca, that is purslane, or ... or sempervive, that is rhubarb, which are all reflective, be added to the aforesaid, the soothing of the pain will be more marked; for in whatever manner they may act they soothe the heated matter and appease the fever of it if applied as a poultice. Should burning heat befall, squill infused in cold water with boniface and applied with a dressing of linen will be found to be curative.

In lippitudo and watery eye, if the patient be aged and decrepit, this ointment best cures: many times have I proved this: which is thus made: use a basin of brass, well greased with fresh butter, and let it stand overnight; in the morning let the basin be inverted upon a pot or dish in which is the sour urine of a man, warmed that it may receive the most urine; let the butter be liquified and when cool take down the basin and thus let it be allowed to stand for a whole day; afterwards let the butter be scraped out, it will appear green, and mix with it a little lard of a capon liquified by the sun's heat or at the fire and store it up in a waxed vessel. Let the eyelid be well anointed. Do not let it run down into the eyes; the eyes should be bandaged, and thus let him lie all night. Of a surety let it be dissolved in the morning, but not washed, then it will be healthy. Again be sure that it is washed with warm water but never with cold. And be it known for certain that by frequent ablution with the proper urine those suffering from festered or punctured wounds may be . . . and gritty feelings and continual debility of the sight can be improved. For truly everything referred to above deletes, comforts, strengthens and preserves, especially from lippitudo.

This medicine was highly beneficial to my own eyes in studying and writing until the seventieth year of my age; much having been undertaken.

And know all men present and to come that I Master John of Ardern and the least of surgeons wrote this little book painfully with my own hand at London in the first year of the (?) victorious King Richard the Second and in the seventieth year of my age.

And if anyone consider this medicine to be common and of no value he may take heed that I have cured very many with it in my time. God knows who cures, not myself. But it is known that the urine should not be fresh but a little acid, that is of the age of two days in summer and three in winter, and if the urine be injected in the basin as enjoined it will be very effectual, if used the following morning; whereas fresh urine breeds worms in the hands and eyelids if they are bathed with it. With this medicine and by the use of fennell seeds a man should be able to cure himself of blindness and pains, as I have proved unless he be of a jaundiced disposition, without any other medicine. And after the ablution with urine the sufferers should bathe the face and eyelids, the eyes being closed, with warm water and dry with a cloth. Oriental crocus being dried upon a warm towel and powdered, and then digested with white of egg beaten up may be instilled into the eyes, the clearest part of it being used. Again having closed the eye place on it a poultice of yolk of a raw egg and crocus aforesaid prepared upon a dressing made of fine linen. It draws out the redness from the eyes and is wonderful for macula. If one or two drops of natural balsam be instilled into an eye with pannus or macula two or three times it purges well and not too sharply; it makes the sight acute and preserves it in its natural virtue, and this I have proved no less by myself as by many others; which balsam I have always ready at hand.

In the final paragraphs of his treatise Arderne leaves the eye and treats of general matters; laxatives, an acid drink made from danewort and elder pounded with the fat of an old hog and not fired; if burnt aloes be added and again not heated an ointment will result which can be kept for use. This should be rubbed into the lower abdomen; it reduces piles and cures dropsy. Then follows Friar Gordon's method of manufacture taken from his *Lilium*; this consists of a regular blunderbuss of about twenty-two ingredients, a full teaspoonful of the mixture to be given in red wine warm. Lastly he gives the manufacture of a trochiscus which is reckoned good for the liver, dry cough and consumption of the body; the trochiscus contains eleven ingredients.

Lotions containing zinc, which are so much used at the present day, can be compared with the famous eye remedy of the Middle Ages, tutty, *i.e.* the crude oxide of zinc.

It is interesting to find Arderne giving the names of some of the herbs he recommends in the vernacular; smallache and red berry crops for instance. Eyebright does not seem to have come into its own as an eye remedy at his date; and most of his herbs are to be found in use in Anglo-Saxon ophthalmology. "God knows who cured him, not myself" reminds us of Ambroise Pare's favourite sentiment of a later date.

Ecclesiastical records such as the bishop's registers occasionally give us an item of ophthalmic interest. One extract from the publications of the Cantilupe Society, which has printed the registers of the Bishops of Hereford, may be allowed in this place as the date is an early one. On September 6th, 1322, Adam Orleton, Bishop of Hereford, gave permission for Robert, Vicar of Fownhope, to resign and be admitted to any other living in the diocese in spite "of the defect which is very apparent in the pupil of one of your eyes". Can this have been a case of coloboma iridis?

The end of the sixteenth century saw the publication of two small ophthalmic books; one of these was Walter Bayley's *A Briefe Treatise touching the preseruation of the Eye-sight*, and the other a translation of Guillemeau's *Maladies de l'Oeil*.

The second of these works was later republished by Richard Banister, and until recently our knowledge of these books was in a state of confusion. This has now been cleared up by Arnold Sorsby.*

To take the second book first, we find that it is a very scarce work. Sorsby has found four copies; two at the Royal Society of Medicine, one at the Medical Society of London and one in the Cambridge University Library. The College of Surgeons and the British Museum do not possess copies and it is not listed in the Surgeon-General's Catalogue. There were two issues. In the first the identity of the translator is disclosed upon the title-page, but unfortunately the name has been erased with ink at some time. After the ink had been washed out the name did not show clearly, but Sorsby hazarded the opinion that it was "A. Hunton". In the second issue the initials "A. H." appear instead of the name. The date of publication is not given but search at Stationers' Hall by Sorsby has narrowed the date to within the years 1585 and 1589. As the book is a translation from the French I do not propose to say anything about the contents. Search by Sorsby and myself has made it practically certain that the translator was A. Hunton. The book is dedicated to "his louing friend Mr John Banester, Chirurgian", the "neare and deare" kinsman who appears in Richard Banister's preface in 1622. At the time of publication John Banester was living at Nottingham and the dedication is from "E. M. in N."; Sorsby suggests that this is East Markham near Retford. An account of Anthony Hunton has been contributed to the Thoresby Society,

* Sorsby, *British Journal of Ophthalmology*, vol. XVI, 1932.

Miscellanea, in 1925, vol. XXVIII, p. 212, by W. J. Kaye. Hunton appears to have been born about 1560 of poor parents. A boy of the same name was admitted a chorister of Southwell Minster in 1574.* Venn, in *Alumni Cantabrigienses,* vol. II, gives "Hunton, or Humpton, Anthony. Matric. sizar from Christ's, June 1575; B.A. 1578–9; M.A. 1582. Licensed to practise medicine, 1589". If he was in practice at East Markham when he published his translation, he must have left soon after. The Notts. Subsidy Roll for 1593 shows him to be, at that date, of Newark-on-Trent. Hunton was acquainted with Gerard, the author of the *Herbal,* and contributed some verses to it. In 1606 Hunton was nominated by James the First lecturer in medicine at Gresham College, but was not elected. He died at Newark in 1624 and was buried there on December 24th. He appears to have been a bachelor; and at the time of his death to have been possessed of a considerable property. The Notts. Final Concords give the details of four fines for the conveyance of land in Newark, Newark and Northgate, Kelham, all in Notts., and in Lincs. at Castroppe, Denton and Barrowby, all near Grantham. His will is preserved at the York Probate Registry, it is dated July 31st, 1624, and was proved by the executor, Samuel Hunton, February 1st, 1624 (O.S.). His brother was Ornan Hunton, and all his nephews rejoiced in such Biblical names as Mordecai, etc.

Among his other activities he did much to popularise Harrogate as a health resort.

WALTER BAYLEY

Walter Bayley was the son of Henry Bayley, of Warnwell, Dorset, and was born at Portsham in the same county. He was elected a scholar of Winchester in 1544† and proceeded to New College, Oxford, in the customary way. After two years at Oxford he was admitted a fellow of New College. He became M.B. 1557; M.D. 1563 and was admitted to practise in 1558.

---

* James, W. A., *Southwell Grammar and Song Schools,* 1927.
† Kirby, *Winchester Scholars.*

About this time he became Prebendary of Dulcote, at Wells, which preferment he held till 1579. In 1561 he became Regius Professor at Oxford and, later, physician to Queen Elizabeth. He was admitted Fellow of the College of Physicians in 1581, was named an Elect in 1584 and Consiliarius in 1588. He died March 3rd, 1592, aged 63, and was buried in New College Chapel, where there is an inscription to his memory. He was the author of several works, and he and his works are the subject of one of Sir D'Arcy Power's admirable papers, which appeared in the *Medico-Chirurgical Transactions*, vol. XC, p. 415.

His little book on the eye is entitled: *A Briefe Treatise touching the Preseruation of the Eiesight, consisting partly in Good Order of Diet and partly in Use of Medicines*. The title-page does not contain either the name of the author or printer, but Sir D'Arcy's copy has an inscription at the end of the preface: "your very lovinge fryende Walter Bayley, 1586". It would appear to have been privately printed for distribution among his friends. As the title-page indicates, the way to keep good sight is to be careful of air and in diet; amongst medicines, euphrasy or eyebright, taken in beer, is extolled. The value of tinted glasses is also mentioned. There were many reprints. Sir D'Arcy finds a sixth edition, edited by Joseph Barnes, at Oxford in 1602, while Munk's *Roll* gives a duodecimo edition of 1616. Sir D'Arcy was not able to find evidence of any editions between the first and the sixth. He gives the transcript of Bayley's long and interesting will and states that he lived, when in London, in Salisbury Court, Fleet Street.

CHAPTER VI

The Seventeenth Century

DURING the seventeenth century the healing art was gradually becoming emancipated from the beliefs of the Middle Ages; and ophthalmology became more practical and less indebted to astrology, spells and charms than previously. We have seen in the last chapter that small books dealing with the eye and eyesight were beginning to be published. Before this the most widely used textbook in use in Europe was the tract by Benevenutus Grassus of Jerusalem, the first edition of which was published in 1474. This has recently been translated and published with a scholarly preface by Dr Casey A. Wood, of Pasadena.

Early in the seventeenth century the composite book by Richard Banister made its appearance; the later years saw the rise of Turberville, Briggs and Coward, of whom the two latter published books, while the former had a great reputation as a clinician. Each of these men was properly qualified.

The most famous ophthalmic condition of the century is the blindness of John Milton. This subject has been most ably dealt with by Arnold Sorsby in a paper in the *British Journal of Ophthalmology* in July 1930. I have his permission to make use of his material in this chapter. It is very unlikely that further evidence on this subject will ever be forthcoming; and as there has been a good deal of misconception in the past about it, Milton's blindness deserves a note in any history of ophthalmology in England.

Briefly, the most favoured conditions which have been suggested to account for Milton's blindness are glaucoma, retinal detachment and choroido-retinal degeneration leading to optic atrophy, the last possibly due to congenital syphilis; while

Mutschmann, a *littérateur*, and not a medical man, has postulated that Milton was an albino, though he accepts Hirschberg's verdict that the blindness was due to glaucoma. The evidence is obtained from autobiographical details in the sonnet to Milton's blindness, in that addressed to his pupil, Syriack Skynner, in *Paradise Lost*, the *Defensio Secunda* and the letter to Philaras. When Stern, in 1879, wrote his life of Milton, he approached "a distinguished ophthalmologist", who stated that "some of the features tended to a diagnosis of glaucoma, though others were against such a view". Hirschberg and Shastid accepted the glaucoma theory without giving reasons. The source is in the letter to Philaras, where Milton states that if he "looked at a lit candle, a kind of iris seemed to snatch" it from him. His sight began to fail in the outer field of the left eye when he was thirty-five years old and he was quite blind by the age of forty-three. Dufour, of Lausanne, argued, in 1909, in favour of retinal detachment complicating myopia. Aubarat and Cabannes, in 1924, postulated congenital syphilis. Milton's eyes were normal to outward appearance after he had been three years blind, as we learn from the Skynner sonnet. The "iris" is the only symptom in favour of glaucoma; while the "copious light glittering from shut eyes" and the description of micropsia and metamorphopsia and the loss of field are far more suggestive of retinal detachment than of glaucoma. There is no reason to take the hypothesis of congenital syphilis seriously; and we can agree with Sorsby's summing-up in favour of retinal detachment.

Another case of ophthalmic trouble in a well-known man in this century is that of Samuel Pepys. Pepys, of course, did not become blind, but he suffered so severely from eyestrain that he had to discontinue his diary at an early age and was incapacitated from work. I have dealt with Pepys's ophthalmic troubles in the *British Journal of Ophthalmology*, vol. v. My view is that, as he was under forty years of age when he gave up his diary, the most likely condition was a low grade of hypermetropic astigmatism, complicated by muscular insufficiency.

Before discussing the men and books of this century I give transcripts of certain manuscripts preserved at the British Museum, which were copied for me by Mr Harvey Bloom. The letter from John Symcotes appeared in the *British Journal of Ophthalmology* for July 1932; so far as I am aware the others have not been published before.

Add. MS. 29244, fol. 10.

Good Mr Powers,

Because this affect proceedes from accidentall distemper rather than any naturall affluxion of humour, it had bene good to have opened a veyne, but nether y^r yeares nor y^s time of ye yeare are propitious, therefore if you find any disordered heates, I advise you to ye use of barly water made with liquerice anise seedes etc. I have directed you four thinges none not physicall as (y^t word is comonly taken) but only to rectify y^r serous humour & voyd it by urine wch is ye intention of ye pills to be taken at nights. I love no much tampering with thinges blowne into ye eye *but now white sugar candy used as you mention can do no hurt.* Therefore you may be bold wth it. I heare y^{or} Dr there is much offended w^t me for . . .ying a^{gt} him. I pray stop ye rumor I assure you I have bene ever silent in ye censure of wandering practitionours & so of him, but for a few words I inserted into a lettre to you, I suffre such to weary out themselves. I think him worthy of contempt not of opposition wch would make the world thinke there were something good in him y^t might disadvantage me. Let him therefore not think of me, as I doe not of him, being neither sorry for his stay, nor glad for removall. This in haste wth my fond love to you I rest,

y^{or} very loving friend

JOHN SYMCOTTES.

Remember my service to Mrs Willis. Dec: 20. 1636.

Bathe y^{or} eyelidd, wth the water in the glasse oftentymes in the day, at y^r pleasure and now and then you may dropp a dropp or 2 into y^r eye especially to bedward and every night to bedward swallow doune 2 of the pills in the boxe, and soe rest.

And every morning fasting, and also about halfe an houre after meales, eate soe much of the powder in the paper as you can take up wth a shillinge.

Alsoe use y^{or} w^{te} ointment yet somtymes, as before.

The writer of this letter was admitted, as John Symcotes, pensioner, at Queens' College, Cambridge, April 1608. He was the son of John Simcotes, of Sutton, Beds. The son matriculated in 1610 and took his B.A. in 1611/12; M.A. in 1615; and his M.D., from King's College, in 1636. His brother, who was also at Cambridge, became a parson and was Rector of a parish in Bedfordshire. The annotation notes are from Venn's *Alumni Cantabrigienses*, vol. IV. I have not been able to find out when Dr Symcotes died.

SLOANE MS. 3801 (BRITISH MUSEUM)

This manuscript consists of a small quarto volume composed partly of narrative and partly of prescriptions. Most of the latter are in the handwriting of the author of the narrative, but some of them are in other handwritings. No author's name is appended to the manuscript. The museum authorities consider it to be of the time of Charles the First and Mr Harvey Bloom dates it between 1630 and 1640. He states that the script is one of the most difficult to decipher that he has ever seen.

This manuscript shows clearly the manners and customs of itinerant quacks; and perusal of the Chevalier Taylor's life proves that their methods were the same in his day.

The narrative part of the manuscript is as follows:

f. 1. Definitions.

f. 2. A Breefe discourse of ye chefeste Oculistes that have bene in this lande or is at this day with theire manner of lyfe and practise to my knowledge.

The firste and chefeste was Luke of Erithe a man that lived in greate fame and credite had the greateste practise and sumes of money for he hathe had from xx to lx l for Cataracke couchinge.

f. 2 d. He keepte those that had theire Cataracke couched close for ix dayes to ly in new bedes & upon theire backes. He got verye muche by a dyet drinke he used ffor moste diseeses he v'sed London everye year'e He neuer set upe bils that I heard of but those that desyred his helpe & dwelled far from him he would appoynte a tyme to come to them and would wyshe ym to gyve notis of his cominge to alle they knewe stoode in need of his helpe.

f. 3. He grewe ryche and bylded a fayre house. He left one sonne behind him who had no skill so that all his knowledge was buryed wth him. He died at London at Mr Bests house in ye stockes.

Then ther was one Mr Surphlete a man of axeolente Dyet and crusty fasion of bodye. He lived till he was fouere score yeares of age lived moste in Norfolke & dyed at Linn and in good estate. He lay 2 or 3 yeares at a barber's house at Linn to whom he taught som skille, who nowe professethe it wth weak Understandinge and gyven to drinke I cannot com'end this Mr Surphlete for any extra-ordinarye skille though of longe experience.

Then was their one Mr Barnaby of Peterborough an honeste and religious man & a good oculiste & resonable surgeon.

f. 4. All these used one order in their practise.

Then was their one Earle in Staffordshire a good artiste I can speake no further of him.

Then was their on Henry Blackburne who travelled contynuouslye from one market towne to another, who could couche ye Cataracke welle, cure yt, Laye a scar Lipe, set a crockt necke strayght & helpe deafnesse.

f. 4. Though he could doe good in these cures yet he was soe wickedlye gyven that he would cousen & deceave men of great som of moneys by taken incurable diseases in hand. He was lusty amorously gyven to seueral women so that his coseninge made him fearfully to flee from place to place & often changed his name and habits in divers places, & was often imprisoned for women. His skille was excelente, but his vices . . . *longus*, his practeste was this, yf he made a blinde man see; after he had couched ye Cataracke and he

f. 5. . . . prepare ye Lady. He dubled a thicke linen clothe wet in ye white of an ege beaten, & so gave him divers lianst to dresse ye eyes twyce a daye for ix dayes together & so he lefte ym, yf he herde they did welle he woulde see ym agayne, yf not he would neuer come at ym. If cum payne or accedentlyes fell out they receaved no com-forte from him.

f. 5 d. When he set a croked necke strayghte where two synowes were to be cut he thruste ye sharpe knyfe under bothe ye synowes nere ye necke ye edge outworde & so cut ye synowes asunder & cut ye skin cleane throughe than he made a tent put in *ott. rosarum* & so dressed it up laying for that lyve Kole . . . & ye whit of an ege, then wyshed tham—dressinge to cut ye tents shorter or rype it & yf it in ye most cases till he was whole.

f. 6. Though before I com'ended him for a good oculist it was for his manuel operation & not his method or medicines. He dyed in Kent after he had thoroughly travelled alle partes of the lande, he left no memorie of his gaynes or gettinges his wicked lyfe was suche that I thinke he had not one friend that he trusted, but alwayes that he got he caryed about with him. He was often deceaued of great sums of money yet neuer robbed.

f. 6 d. He dyed but in meane estate had one sonne and left him nothing That I pray Goad alle good oculists may be warned by him to walke uprightly in their callinge to lyve in ye feare of God and then theye are sure to die so for *QUALIS VITA I'T'NIS ITAR* This Blackburne did instructe one Page and Hanle

Page was a pothecary then sett in his practise but neuer was experte.

f. 7. nor neuer wilke he is of large stature, a large harte, & a shakinge hande.

Blackburne instructed one Nelson that maryed his sister. he could couche the Cataracke welle but was gyven to drunkeness & so dyed beggarly.

Nowe I can speak of Hanle whom Blackburne firste taughte. he hath an able bodye, hath travelled moste partes of Englande as his tutor did and great stryfe was betwixte them wch should have the greater practise and since he was muche infected with his tutors qualetys, as many times he would take money where noe good was to be done. he would deale wth moste Catarackes whether they were redye or noe. make ym see for ye present get money, put ye reste to adventure, by wch meanes he did banishe himselfe from many places where he cam & neuer durste come their againe.

f. 8. & for his deceipt was once beaten by a gentleman and often threatened, troubled, & in danger by his ungodlye & synister dealing, Yet I neuer knewe that he changed his name, but in some places would not make himselfe knowne, his fassyon was to spende franklye in his Innes, in Allhowses, & tauernes, so got his fame & acquaintances. he would neuer stay in a place where he had couched Cataracts, till their eyes were opened but traueled in haste and sayde he (was)

f. 8 d. trauelinge to som greate ladye knighte or suche like. The course wherof was yf ye patient did not see after nyne dayes they would look for restitution backe agayne, yf ye patiente fell into payne he could use no meanes to ease ym, for he had no learninge at all, nor could he discribe any disease by his name but sayde wher he meant to deale honestlye all diseases were outworkes excepte for these that he thus delte wth

f. 9. If they have Inflamtion or Reumes in their eyes he wold alwayes have a pewter kettle wth water wherein was put white wine rose water & Camphire wthout proportion or mesure, of that water he woulde gyve a little glasse fulle & take a 5s or 6s as he could get for it. To those that had watering eyes or sighte decayinge, the eyes moyste or dry, he would often tyme stiche ym & get 4 or V li as he could get by

f. 9 d. that meanes. For couchinge of Cataracke he would do it exelente welle, his order was after he had couched ym, to dype large & thicke pledgethe of towe in a sponefulle or twoe of Sallet oyle with oyle of Roses yf he had it & then dype it ageyne in ye white of an ege in reason & so close ym upe & so to contynuance for 3 dayes, & the 3d daye agayne to soe dresse ym, then ye nexte nighte

f. 10. to take alle from theire eyes in ye nighte, and this was (it) he used for his easening drinke wth seuen soles sugar (?) etc. For other diseases, whiche modestye. . . conceale of, his manner of boastinge was he could doe as muche under God for ye eyes as alle the men in Englande, & for ye eyes he would dispute wth the Universities of Oxforde & Cambridge, or with many other Vayne Empiricall Prostestations wch he dayly used whersoeuer he came

f. 10 d. He got muche especyally Brother Blackburne's cursonage, and his was knowne in euery place of ye lande What siluer he got he would change as muche as he could into gould, & cary home to his wyfe, who was very constantly gyven & would carefully keepe what he got. he had no children nor charge but his wyfe & him selfe, so that he could but be richer than many of the other oculists within a fewe yeares. At

f. 11. his firste beginninge he came to Sleaforde wher I dwelled, & their in ye market set upe his showe or pictures, & made proclama-tion where I grew acquainted wth him & after wth Mr Blackburne at Yorke. Nowe I leave them & com to discourse particularly & trulye of my selfe My firste meanes & methode of practise & breeflye of my behaviour in my trauels and of my successe therin.

f. 11 d. Firste for my Education I was broughte upe as a gramar scoler in the countrye & after I had learned from part of Tullyes Offyces & som other lating books, but no vearse or poetrye. My father sent my brother Gabriell & my yonger brother to be a prentise with my Uncle, he was youthfullye gyven went (the) Portingal Voyage, & dyed there I had another yonger brother called John, he

PLATE III

was bound an apprentise wth a barber surgeon He dyed of ye sicknes

It pleased God to spare & reserve me to be educated & instructed wth my Uncle 5 or 6 yeares in ye practise of surgerye atte ye tyme I was wth him I euer collected what receiptes I could get & carefully observed alle practise. then I wayted a yeare or twoe of ye Lorde Willaby in his chamber. then I spent a little tyme (with) one James of Utricke in ye Lowe Cuntryes. (vide illustration.)

f. 12 d. Then I retourned and settled myselfe at Sleaforde where I lived welle for fourtene yeares and carefullye & studiouslye practisinge surgerye, and studyed muche my Uncles booke of Anathomy, of ye nutritive & natural partes, wch was greate credite untoe me for no Surgeon or few Doctors were able to reason wth me in those partes & I had divers good books of surgerye which I dayly (had) recourse to as occasion was

f. 13. offered in my practise For when eney wast wounded I perused euery authors judgement & for other diseases so tha i was alwayes able by reason of my skill to discharge a good conscience sincere as good & gyve good satisfaction to my patientes & their friendes, wch was great credite & comforte unto me, besyde I made alle my medicines my selfe & would bestowe (them) furnyshed upon alle sodayne occasions then all ye

The narrative ends abruptly, the verso being in another hand and containing a Latin prescription.

The author takes some credit to himself for being a "gramar scoler". No doubt he compared favourably with the itinerant quacks of the Blackburne type.

It is a pity he did not give his name; it will be noticed that he had brothers named Gabriel and John and that he was trained by his uncle. May I suggest that the writer may have been a son of Richard Banister and that the uncle with whom he studied may possibly have been John Bannester, Richard's "neare and deare kinsman"?

Among the manuscripts at the British Museum is a small treatise (Sloane MS. 1187) written on forty-six paper pages. It is probably of the date of Charles the Second. This little volume is lettered on the back: "Buckley De Affectib. Oculor. et Aurium". The first thirty-six pages are occupied by closely written notes on diseases of the eye. There is a preface and eighteen short chapters which include remarks on gutta serena, affections of the vitreous and crystalline, of the aqueous and "chiefly suffusion", on dilated and contracted pupils, on albugo, ophthalmia, hypopyon, phlyctenules, corneal ulcers, cancer of the cornea, rupture of the cornea, prolapse of the uvea, lacrymal conditions, epiphora and pterygium.

Such portions of this book as I have seen appear to be commonplace; the text is in Latin throughout.

The author would appear to be Thomas Buckley, M.D. I do not know where he graduated. He seems to have been rather a prolific author of manuscript medical works and there are several of these in the British Museum. It is possible that the Buckley who went out to China and was a correspondent of the Royal Society is the man in question. He appears to have sent a present of some china to the King, and Sir Hans Sloane was commissioned to write and thank him.

RICHARD BANISTER

Banister's book was thought at one time to be the earliest separate and complete work on ophthalmology in the English tongue. That this view is no longer tenable has been ably demonstrated by Arnold Sorsby. Actually the book is a collection of five separate treatises comprising 478 unnumbered pages. Of these the first 112 pages are Banister's own contribution to the book; this is named Banister's breviary. The bulk of the book following the breviary is an unacknowledged translation of Guillemeau's *Maladies de l'Oeil*, introduced by a separate title-page. The third section, of thirty pages, is an unacknowledged reprint of Walter Bayley's *A Briefe Treatise concerning the Preseruation of the Eye-Sight.* Then follow two pages of introduction and a "Discourse of the Scorby"; and lastly thirty-four pages on the "Nature and Divers Kinds of Cancers or Cankers"; the first of which is translated out of "Wyer's Observations", and

the second, "painfully weaved by Textor". The latter gentleman would appear to be the "A. H.", the translator of Guillemeau's treatise. The book was published in 1622; the breviary
being dated from Stamford, "the last day of Iune, 1621".

Banister makes it quite clear that "The Treatise, etc." is "the
second time published". In his dedication "To the Reader", he
draws attention to the fact that he here publishes "the labours
of a worthy writer ——— who describeth an hundred and
thirteene severall diseases happening to the eyes and eielids, with
their particular causes, symptomes, signes and cures; the worke
was dedicated to my forenamed kinsman (John Banester), and
being long since out of print, it is not now to be bought for
money; and this booke have I sent abroade againe, that those
which delight to labour in this Art, may runne the readier way
to the better successe. I have also added something of mine
owne, that through my experience they may finde at first, what I
was learning long".

As Sorsby says, the book is obviously the work of an honest
man and a careful observer. In the breviary a discussion on
gutta serena appears after the verses on "The fit time for
couchi(ng) of Cataracts". Banister lays emphasis upon the
seriousness of gutta serena; he had only two successes, and many
failures, in his treatment of this condition. He goes on to say:
"When it pleaseth God to inable my skill, that I understand a
more perfect Cure for this dangerous disease, I will publish the
meanes that are most effectual and approved, whereby the
Practitioner and the Patient may be the lesse mistaken in their
expectation, but according to my observation, I will show my
opinion, where most hope of Cure is: if the humour settled in
the hollow Nerves, be growne to any solid, or hard substance,
it is not possible to be cured; which may be iudged of, foure
wayes. First, if it be of long continuance. Secondly, if they see
no light at all of the sun, fire or candle. Thirdly, if one feele the
Eye by rubbing upon the Eie-lids, that the Eye be growne more
solid and hard, than naturally it should be. Fourthly, if one per-

ceive no dilatation of the *pupilla*, then there is no hope of Cure. Contrariwise, if the sight hath beene lost but a small time, viz., a moneth or two, if the Eye be perceived soft and pliable, if there be any *dilatio* in *Pupilla*, though it can scarcely be perceived, yet there is some hope of Cure".

This clear recognition of hardness of the eyeball, both as a physical condition, and as a sign of the utmost value in prognosis, is of the greatest importance historically. His remarks fell on stony ground and more than two hundred years were to pass before his teaching became part of the ophthalmic creed.

Banister died in 1626. Although he has been deemed worthy of a place in the *Dictionary of National Biography*, Banister is an elusive person and very little is known about him. A good deal of research, by Arnold Sorsby and myself, has failed to add much to our knowledge of the man. The name is a common one and is spelt in a variety of ways, *e.g.* Banister, Bannister, Banester, Banastre. We have not been able to establish his parentage; and beyond a reference in the *History of Stamford* (Peck), and the details of his will, we have little to add to what is already known about him. It is a pity in many respects, for he deserves well of ophthalmology and has received scanty justice at our hands.

In the *History of Stamford*, among the list of "benefactors to St Maries Parish", occurs the following statement: "Mr Richard Banister late of the same parish, gent. erected at his owne costs and charges in the South Quire, a publick library, and gave some books to the same, as Galens works, and some other books both of physick and chyrurgery. And at his death gave £10 in money the interest of which summe is yeerly to be bestowed in books for the increase of the said library, such as the minister of that his parish shall think most fit". A footnote states that only a few shelves and a partition were put up, and that the money is "now" lost.

LINCOLN CONSISTORY COURT, 1626, fol. 496

Testator

RICHARD BANISTER of STAMFORD in the County of Lincoln,
gent.

Will dated

4th April, 2nd year King Charles, 1626.
To be buried in the South Choir in the parish Church in St Marys
in Stamford.

Bequests

To the said Parish Church ten pounds to be put forth by the
Minister and Churchwardens at the rate of seven pounds in the
hundred and the interest bestowed upon Divinity Books
yearly, or once in two years, and such books to be placed in the
Library of the said Parish Church and there to remain for ever.

To Gabriell Banister, my eldest son, twenty marks of lawful
English money and also "Garratts Herbal together with my
vellet bagg wch I used to weare in my travell & my box of
silver instruments".

To Richard Banister, my second son, ten pounds and my porte-
mantue.

To John Banister, my third son, five pounds at his age of twenty
two.

To my said sons Gabriell and Richard "all my other English books
(being Physick & Surgerie & not Divinitie), boxes, bottles,
glasses as they are furnished to be equally divided betwixt
them provided that my Will is that my sonn Gabriell shall have
his cheyce".

To Francis Banister, my fourth son, all my Latten Books in the
Chest, in the shopp and in the little bord chest in the Chamber
with the manuscript books in the same and fifty pounds to be
paid at his age of twenty one, my son Richard to have the
keeping of my son Francis his books, giving my Executors
security for the same.

To Brigett Banister, my eldest daughter, fifty pounds at her age
of twenty years and also my first wife's riding cloak, safeguard
and hood and her best stuff gown laced with gold and silver
lace and one of my greatest trunks to put her clothes in.

To Susan Banister, my youngest daughter, fifty pounds at her age of twenty years and my middle nest of boxes as they are furnished with my bagg and the lignum vitæ in the same and also one of my biggest trunks.

To my said daughters Brigett and Susan all my English books of Divinitie to be equally divided betwixt them.

To Brigett Lupton, widow, twenty shillings for her care and pains she hath heretofore taken with my former wife in the time of her sickness.

To Elizabeth Banister, my loving wife, all the goods and chattels that were hers before our intermarriage and also all my other goods and chattels within the realm of England (not given or bequeathed heretofore by me).

To my said Wife, Elizabeth Banister and X'pofer Manninge of Stamford aforesaid, Shoomaker, and their heirs for ever, my freehold land lying in Stamford Barron and in the Fields thereof in the County of Northampton in the tenure of John Yeomens or his assigns with a sure trust and confidence I have in them that they will sell the same and the moneys accrueing to them for the same shall be for and towards the payment of my debts and legacies.

𝕰𝖝𝖊𝖈𝖚𝖙𝖔𝖗𝖘

My said wife Elizabeth Banister and the said X'pofer Manninge.

𝖂𝖎𝖙𝖓𝖊𝖘𝖘𝖊𝖘

Richard Langton Timothie Evat. Em. Com'.

(The date of probate is not shown.)

A search of the Bishops' Transcripts of Stamford, St Mary's Parish Register, kindly conducted by Canon C. W. Foster, revealed the following facts: "Francis Banister, baptised December 10th, 1615. Francis (*sic*) daughter of Richard Banister, buried March 27th, 1619. On Ladyday 1623, 1624 Richard Banister signs as churchwarden. Ann, 'ye wife of Richard Banister, gent.', buried April 16th, 1624. Richard Banister, gentleman, buried April 7th, 1626. George Freeman and Bridget Banister, married August 24th, 1627. Christopher Banister, 'ye sonne of Gabriell Banister, Chirugian', baptised November 29th, 1629."

TURBERVILLE OF SALISBURY

This memoir deals with a man who belongs to an early age in English ophthalmology, the seventeenth century, when medicine generally was only just emerging from the astrological period. It is a remarkable fact that he was not only a properly qualified medical man, but also a member of an ancient English family; records of which go back to the days of King John, if not earlier still; and branches of which were settled in various counties. The name would appear to have been adapted by Thomas Hardy in his *Tess of the D'Urbervilles*. John Durbeyfield, when boasting of his ancestors in the church at Kingsbere and saying: "There's not a man in the county of South-Wessex that's got grander and nobler skillentons in his family than I", is presumably referring to the Turbervilles of Bere Regis in Dorset. Mr Hardy is in error in making Parson Tringham state that "their names appear in the Pipe rolls in the time of King Stephen", for there is a sad break in the series of these rolls from the last of Henry the First to the second of Henry the Second; and the rolls for Stephen's reign, if they ever existed, are no longer among the Public Records of the Kingdom.

Dawbigney Turberville, the subject of these notes, was a son of George Turberville, gent., of Wayford, co. Somerset. In Collinson's *History* of that county will be found quite a number of early references to the Turberville family; thus, William de Turberville was Sheriff of the county in 1256-7; Sir Richard de Turberville, Sheriff, 1356-7; Sir John de Turberville, Sheriff, 1487; while Henry de Turberville, in the seventeenth of King John, had wardship of Nicholas FitzMartin of Chewton; and William de Turberville, in the fifteenth of Henry the Sixth, was holding a third part of the manor of Moreton in the same county. In the forty-seventh of Edward the Third, Cicely Beauchamp of Shepton-Beauchamp married, as her second husband, Richard Turberville of Bere Regis, and bore on her seal "checky", the arms of Turberville. In the *Testa de Nevill* the name will be found in connexion with the counties of Hereford, Warwick, Leicester and Berkshire.

Dawbigney was of Oriel College, Oxford, matriculating November 7th, 1634, aged 19 years. He took his B.A. October 15th, 1635; his M.A. July 17th, 1640; and his M.D. August 7th, 1660.* We next hear of him serving as a combatant for the King at the siege of Exeter in 1646. When the city was captured by Fairfax he quitted the military life and settled at Wayford.

The chief account of Dr Turberville is to be found in Walter Pope's *Life of Seth Ward, Bishop of Salisbury*, 1697. In this scarce book a whole chapter (number 16, of Dr Turbervile) is devoted to our Salisbury oculist, and from it I have abstracted most of what follows in a somewhat abridged form. Turberville cured the writer, Pope, who says: "It was he who twice rescued me from blindness, which without his aid had been unavoidable, when both my eyes were so bad, that with the best I could not perceive a letter in a book, not my hand with the other, and grew worse and worse every day".

Turberville was born in 1612 of an old-English family, "there being in the church of Beer only, the tombs of no less than fifteen Knights of that name, as I have been credibly informed, but I confess I have not seen them". His mother was a Dawbigney, and it was upon her advice, according to Pope, that the son took up the study of eye diseases at the University.

While besieged at Exeter he and a friend ran in debt £100 each, "in chalk behind the door; he told me that his landlord came into their chamber, leading his daughter by the hand, and courteously proffered to cancel the debts of either of us who should marry her". Turberville "valiantly resisted this temptation and chose rather to pay his debts in ready money, which he did shortly after; the other accepted the terms, and has his wife's portion presently paid him, *viz.*, his scores wiped out with a wet dishclout".

The articles allowed the garrison of Exeter to return to their

* Foster's *Alumni Oxonienses*, 1st series, vol. IV.

dwellings; Turberville went to Wayford and married, but had no children. He began practice at Wayford and Crookhorn (Crewkerne), but got so busy that he moved to London. The city air not suiting him he finally settled in Salisbury; "thence he made several journeys to London. Once he was sent for by the Dutchess of York to cure the Princess of Denmark (Queen Anne), then a child, labouring under a dangerous inflammation in her eyes, and a breaking out in her face the cure for which had been attempted in vain by the Court fysicians". These despised Turberville, looking on him as a country quack. He had a quarrel with them, refused to meet them in consultation and won the day. The Duke and Duchess asked him to undertake the case, which he did successfully. The Duke ordered him a fee of £600, but he appears to have received only half that amount. "Many years afterwards he was called up again by one of the greatest and ancientest Peers of this Kingdom, to whom, after having attentively inspected his eye, he spoke after this manner: 'My Lord, I might bear you in hand', a western frase, signifying to delay or keep in expectation, 'and feed you with promises, or at least hopes, that I should cure you in some competent time, and so cause your Lordship to be at great expence to no purpose; I cannot cure you, and I believe no man in England can'. The Earl answered, 'Such and such will undertake it for a hundred pounds'. To which the doctor replied, 'I have so great an honour for your Lordship, and so much wish for your welfare, that I will joyfully give a hundred guineas out of my own purse to the person who shall restore your sight in that eye. I confess I am not able to cure it, but I can reduce it to a better figure'."

Turberville was no boaster, "he generally prescribed to all, shaving their heads and taking tobacco, which he had often known to do much good, and never any harm to the eyes. Far from covetous, he cured the poor gratis, and received from others what they pleased to give him, never, that I knew, making any bargain for so much in hand, and the rest when the cure is perfected, as some do". Pope could never force anything on him for his medicines and extraordinary care, unless it were a cane, a tobacco-box or some new book. "He has cured several who were born blind, but I do not look upon that as so great a thing; for the cure of such, if curable, for there are several sorts of cataracts uncurable, consists wholly in this, *viz.*, in knowing when the connate cataract is fit to be couched, in having a steady hand, and skill to perform that operation, to be able to prevent, or at least, remove the pains which usually follow, and sometimes kill the patient; but to reduce fallen and inverted eyelids to their proper place and tone, to cure inveterate ulcers, and inflammations of a blackish colour, requires a consummate artist. *Hic labor, hoc opus est.*"

Patients came from all over the country and even from abroad; one is mentioned from Jamaica; she was cured but died of smallpox before she could return to her home. It was good business for the City of Salisbury; his patients "being lodged in inns and private houses through all quarters of the city: one could scarce peep out of doors, but have a prospect of some led by boys or women, others with bandages over one or both eyes, and yet a greater number wearing green silk upon their faces, a stranger might have reported the air of Salisbury to be as pernicious to the eyes as that of Orleans is to the nerves, where almost one-third of the inhabitants are lame".

Tales of two patients are next related. In one, a countryman with a bloodshot eye consulted Turberville, who, after inspection, told the man that the inflamed eye was the better of the two. The man vowed that he could see equally well with either eye, but on the inflamed eye being covered, found that he could see nothing with the other and exclaimed: "I am blind in it, tho' to all the rest who were there, it seemed a good eye". In the second case, a man came with a protuberant eye, which could not be contained within the lids and seemed to be like a piece of raw flesh. Dr Turberville "placed him in a chair and with a pair of scissors cut large gobbetts, the blood trickling down his cheeks in abundance, and yet he seemed no more concerned, than if it had been a barber cutting his hair. I was surprised at his behaviour and said to one of the bystanders, 'without doubt this is a married man otherwise 'twere impossible he should be so patient'; which he overhearing in the midst of his torment burst into a loud laughter, and replied, 'No indeed, I am but a batchelor'".

Dr Turberville left his estate between a niece of his wife's and his sister Mary Turberville, "who now practises in London with good reputation and success. She has all her brother's receipts, and having seen his practice during many years knows how to use them. For my part I have so good an opinion of her skill that should I again be afflicted with sore eyes, which God forbid, I would rely upon her advice rather than upon any pretenders or professors in London or elsewhere".

Dr George C. Peachey has kindly given me a reference to the *London Gazette*, June 5th, 1701, wherein occurs the following advertisement:

Mrs Mary Turberville, sister to the late Dr Turberville of Salisbury, liveth in Little Lincoln's Inn, near the Grange Inn, and practises on diseases curable of the eye.

Lest any should be surprised at Mary Turberville taking on the practice I may remind readers that Sir William Read's widow carried on his business after his death at Durham Yard, Strand.*
Pope's chapter ends as follows:

Adieu my dear friend, a rivederci, till we meet and see one another again with eyes which will never stand in need of a COLLYRIUM.

Appended is the following epitaph:

M.S.

Near this place, lies interred the most expert and successful oculist that ever was, perhaps that ever will be,

DR DAWBIGNEY TURBERVILLE.

Descended from two families of those names, than which there are few more ancient and noble. During the Civil War he bore arms for

* James, R. R. "Sir William Read," *Trans. Ophthal. Soc. of the U.K.* vol. xli, p. 342.

the King. After the surrender of Exeter he lived at Wayford and Crookhorn; but those towns not affording conveniences to his numerous patients he removed to London, intending to settle there, but not having his health he left it and lived in Salisbury more than 30 years, doing good to all, and being beloved by all.

His great fame caused multitudes to flock to him, not only from all parts of this Kingdom, but also from Scotland, Ireland, France, and America. He died April 21st, 1696, in the 85th year of his age. And left his estate betwixt his only sister and niece, at whose expenses this monument was erected.

Doctor Walter Pope wrote this epitaf to perpetuate his gratitude, and the memory of his friend and benefactor.

THE *PHILOSOPHICAL TRANSACTIONS*

In the fourteenth volume of the *Philosophical Transactions*, p. 81, will be found two letters from that experienced oculist, Dr Turberville of Salisbury, to Mr William Musgrave, S.P.C., of Oxon., containing several remarkable cases in physic, relating chiefly to the eyes. The first letter, dated London, August 4th, 1684, runs:

The disease which in some late discourse with you I named bursa oculi or the pouch of the eye, was a bag without matter in it, like an empty purse on the white of the eye under the upper lid. It hung flag about the length of a thumb nail. Another person had no visible disease in his eyes, but could not see at all unless he squeezed his nose with his fingers, or saddled it with narrow spectacles, and then saw very well; him I carried to Mr Boyle as a fit subject for so great a philosopher to make his remarks on.

A maid, 22 or 23 years old, came to me from Banbury, who could see very well but no colour beside black and white. She had such scintillations by night with the appearance of bulls, bears, etc., as terrified her very much; she could see to read sometimes in the greatest darkness for almost a quarter of an hour.

The second letter, dated Sarum, October 5th, 1684, runs:

A saddler's daughter of Burford had an imposthume which broke in the corner of one of her eyes, out of which came about thirty stones, splendid, and as large as pearls.

A person in Salisbury had a piece of iron or steel stuck in the iris of the eye which I endeavoured to push out with a small spatula, but could not; but on applying a loadstone it immediately jumped out.

Another person had for a long time been troubled with a great pain and convulsions in his cheek; you might cover the place where the pain was with a penny; the convulsions drew his mouth, face and eye aside: he had used many things prescribed him by physicians and surgeons, but to no purpose. I applied a cupping glass to the place with fired flax in it; then scarified and cupped him again; after which I put on a plaster of diapalma, and he was perfectly cured. I was consulted by a maid who had a pustule broke in her eye out of which there came fine small sand, like chalk, for many weeks together. By the use of purging, fumigation, and some tonics, she recovered her sight in a very great measure.

In vol. xv, p. 109, will be found some observations on the practice of physic by Dr Turberville, of Salisbury:

A gentlewoman was much troubled with falling sickness; in her water I saw a great number of short worms full of legs, and like millepedes; I gave her two or three purges, first with pil. agaric. and rhubarb, but still perceived in every water that was brought to me eight, ten, or more of the worms. They appeared lively and full of motion, and the fits continued daily. At last I gave her half an ounce of oxymel helleboratum in tansy water, which wrought well and was successful, so that she had a complete cure.

About six or seven years since I had a gent^m. (Mr Oyliff) in cure for his eye, which was as large as my fist, black and fleshy, and full of bluish bladders, this I judged to be a cancer. After bleeding and purging I cut out the ball and ulcered flesh by many cuts, which were all insensible to him, till I came to the optic nerve; at the last cut he complained, and bled a little; the wound was healed in about a fortnight; he now wears a black patch over the place. Not long after this a young man had an eye as large as a hen's egg, very fair, without blemish, rheum, or redness, and his sight was pretty tolerable. I judged these symptoms to proceed from thin humours fallen on the eye and distending its coats. I cured this distemper by applying drying medicines to the head and eyes, and making an issue in nucha. *Appello morbum oculorum bovinum, sive oculi hydropem.*

Turberville deserves to be remembered for his use of the magnet in removing foreign bodies from the eye. Hirschberg* points out that the word iris here does not mean that the foreign body was actually in the globe, but that it was embedded in the cornea at the limbus. Of the other cases described in these letters it is impossible to be sure, but the last case would seem to be a case of buphthalmos, while it has been suggested to me that the thirty stones may conceivably have come from a dermoid. The case of total colour blindness is interesting. I surmise that Mr Oyliff may have had an old staphylomatous eye.†

On June 22nd, 1668, Pepys notes in his diary:

My business was to meet Mr Boyle, which I did, and discoursed about my eyes: and he did give me the best advice he could, but refers me to one Turberville of Salisbury, lately come to town, who I will go to.

June 23, to Dr Turberville about my eyes, whom I met with: and he did discourse, I thought, learnedly about them; and takes time before he did prescribe me anything, to think of it.

June 29, to Dr Turberville's, and there did receive a direction for some physic, and also a glass of something to drop into my eyes: he gives me hopes that I may do well.

July 3, to an alehouse: met Mr Pierce, the surgeon, and Dr Clerke, Waldron, Turberville, my physician for the eyes, and Lowe, to dissect several eyes of sheep and oxen, with great pleasure, and to my great information. But strange that this Turberville should be so great a man, and yet to this day had seen no eyes dissected, or but once, but desired this Dr Lowe to give him the opportunity to see him dissect some.

July 5, about four in the morning took four pills of Dr Turberville's prescribing for my eyes, and I did get my wife to spend the morning reading of Wilkins's Reall Character.

Turberville married Ann, daughter of the Rev. James Ford of Hawkchurch, Dorsetshire; he lies buried in the nave of Salisbury

* Hirschberg, J. *Geschichte der Augenheilkunde*, in *Graefe-Saemisch Handbuch*, vol. XIV, ch. XXIII, p. 118. 1911.

† Dr Ernest Thomson writes to me suggesting that the case of bursa oculi may have been a dacryops or the remains of such a cystic structure.

Cathedral, and has the following inscription on a mural tablet on the west wall; under a shield of arms given below:

S.M.

D'AUBIGNY TURBERVILLE M.D. *et Annae uxoris carissimae*
Haec Stemmate Religione, spectabili progenata
Jacobi Ford Ecclesie de Hawchurch Dorcestriae Comitatu
Pastoris vigilantissimi filia:
Optimo marito uxor optima,
Cui Pietas, Prudentia, aliaeque omnes Virtutes
Pari jure summeque dilecto.
Ille ex utraque Prosapia illustri pariter et antiqua oriundus,
Weyfordiae agro Somersetensi natus
Dei cultor sincerus & assiduus Egenis largus, Universis
Amicus facete comis et beneficus;
Denique grande Probitatis exemplar emicuit;
Caeterum OPTHALMIAE *Scientia adeo praecelluit,*
Ut IPSE, *solus ab omni terrarum parte,*
Pulchre notus fuerit et celebratus
Cujus Fama hoc Marmore perennior nunquam peribit.

	⎰*Haec* XVth *Decembris*	
Naturae	⎟*Anno Aetatis* LXXX	MDCXCIV
Concesserunt	⎟*Ille* XXI *Aprilis*	
	⎱*Anno Aetatis* LXXXV	MDCXCVI

Oh nostram omnium sortem lugendam!
Quali fruebamur dum Enituit vivus
Quanto privamur, cum infra jacet extinctus
Solus oculorum Aesculapius.

The shield of arms is as follows: "ermine, a lion rampant gules crowned or, for Turberville, impaling, per fesse in chief a greyhound courant and in base an owl within a bordure engrailed argent and sable, all countercharged". (N.B. The owl has at some time or other been painted wrongly gold.)

His will was proved in London, May 14th, 1696. The abstract is as follows:

DAWBENEY TURBERVILE of the Close of the Canons of the Cathedrall Church of Sarum, co. Wilts. Doctor in Phisicke. (P.C.C., Bond 82.) June 24, 1695. To be buried in Cathedrall as near my wife as can bee. To Anne Bragg of New Sarum, widow, £150. To Edmund Turbervile liveing near Appothecaries Hall in London, gent. £100. To Sister-in-law, Mary Minterne of Crewkerne, co. Somersett, widow, £100. To Godson Turbervile Bonvile, £100. To the brothers and sisters of said Turbervile Bonvile, £10 each. To ——— Bonvile, spinster, aunt to said Turbervile Bonvile, £20. To Godson Dawbeney Bentley, £10, and one of my largest silver tankards. To Cosen Anne Davies of City of London spinster, £50. To the eldest daughter of Captain James Bale of Crewkerne, £10. To Cosen Mary Davies £10 to buy her mourning. To Robert Sayer, son of Israel Sayer, of the City of London, widow (*sic,* but it presumably means that Israel was dead) and his heirs for ever my right of presentation and advowson of the Church of Weyford near Crewkerne and if he shall be educated at the University of Oxford then to have £50 towards his expenses. To the servants now liveing with me, *viz.*—Christopher Hellyer, Elizabeth Hewlett, and Mary Braden, £10 each if with me when I die. My term of years in a house in Sarum Close leased me by the Vicars Chorall of the Cathedrall to my sister Mary Turbervile of the City of London and to ffrances Davis of the said Close of Sarum and now liveing with me, joyntly and to the longest liver of them. But if after my death the said Mary Turbervile shall ever lodge, harbour or in any manner entertaine either by day or night one named Catherine Eller (or whatever she may be named) formerly liveing in the said Close of Sarum, then the said Mary to have no advantage in her moiety of the said house. To the poor of the Parish of Weyford aforesaid £100 to be laid out in lands. To the Poor of the Close of Sarum (?) to be dispersed amongst them by the Dean and Canons Resident. To the Poor of each Parish of New Sarum, £5. Residue to said Mary Turbervile and ffrances Davis, and they to be executrixes. My friends Thomas Turbervile of Beer Regis, co. Dorset, esqre., Richard Barnaby the elder of Ambersbury, Wilts., gent. and William(?) Burner of Bermeston, Wilts., gent., to be trustees and supervisors to assist said executrixes and for their trouble to have £10 each.

Witnesses: Hampton Jay, Anne Haskett, Mary Davis, John Wells.

The amount at which the estate was sworn is not given; at this date it very rarely is.

Frances Davis married a man named Blackborow, of the Close. She died October 11th, 1716, aged 55 years.

Dr Turberville occupied a house near the St Anne Street Gate, the third house on the north side of the road from it. One of the Canons of Salisbury lives there now; it has a very fine ceiling in the drawing-room with the crest of the Cecils: it is supposed to be the crest of Lord Burleigh.

I cannot offer any probable explanation of the old man's rooted antipathy to Catherine Eller; let us hope that she was only one of his dissatisfied patients. Nor can I account for the two different coats of arms, "checky" in the reign of Edward the Third and as given on the monument. Burke's *General Armory* gives: Ford, of Chagford, Ashburton, Bagtor and Nutwell, co. Devon, supposed by Prince to be descended from Forde of Fordemore in Moreton-Hampstead. Per fesse argent and sable, within a bordure engrailed, in chief, a greyhound courant, in base an owl, all countercharged; while from Papworth's *Ordinary of Armorials* we get: Argent, a lion rampant, gules (among many others). Hugh de Torbervile (A) Harl. MSS. 6137. Turevile (D) Turbervile, (E) de Turbervile, (F) Vandernot, co. Lincoln. The A, D, E, F refer to the rolls in the Harleian MSS. in which the coats are found.

I like to imagine the old man "when the bell till'd, to use the Salisbury frase, to evening prayers", sitting in his seat in the Cathedral, listening to the longwinded sermons of perhaps his friend Bishop Seth Ward, and pondering maybe on some of the illustrious figures of the past connected with the City and Cathedral: of William of the Long Sword, the warrior Earl of Salisbury; and Bishop Roger, the Justiciar, who, on the authority of Bishop Stubbs, owed his rise to favour and his place in the confidence of Henry the First to the expeditious way in which he got through divine service; and wishing probably that his successors in the throne at Salisbury had followed his example in this respect.

In the preparation of this memoir I have been indebted to Miss Targett of Salisbury and to Mr J. J. Hammond, clerk to the Dean and Chapter, for much assistance, particularly to Mr Hammond for references and much local help; to my brother, the hon. librarian of Southwell Cathedral, for the heraldic notes and to Mr Gibbons for the abstract of the will.

WILLIAM BRIGGS, M.D.

Accounts of the work of William Briggs have long been available in Munk's *Roll of the Royal College of Physicians* and in the *Dictionary of National Biography*; but it may not be out of place to notice him as an ophthalmologist of the seventeenth century, a date when qualified ophthalmologists were few and far between.

The Briggs family was of respectable antiquity in East Anglia. The pedigree printed in Blomefield and Parkin's *History of Norfolk* (1808) begins with a William atte Brigge, of Salle, *temp*. Edward the First and Second, and living at Salle in 1334. From this William descended Augustine Briggs, son of Thos. Brygge, Esq., of North Wotton, 1546; whose son, Augustine Briggs, of Norwich, was the father of our ophthalmologist.

Augustine Briggs junior was born in 1617 and died in 1684. His wife's name was Elizabeth Aldred. He was a prominent citizen of Norwich. Elected Alderman in 1660, he was named as one of the Aldermen in the new charter given to the City by Charles the Second in 1663. He was Mayor of Norwich in 1670; and in the year 1667 was elected Burgess of Parliament for the City without opposition. This post of M.P. was retained by him at three subsequent elections. Augustine was a benefactor to the City; for, by his will, he made provision for the Boys' and Girls' Hospital (*i.e.* schools) of the City, and he left a sum of money (£200) to the Mayor and Corporation, the interest on which was to be used yearly for putting two poor boys to convenient trades. These boys were to be chosen from his own ward if possible and in the event of no candidate being forthcoming in any year the interest was to be added to the money in the hanaper (City treasury). William Briggs was his second son. As he was thirteen years of age when he was admitted at Corpus Christi

College, Cambridge, in 1663,* it is obvious that he must have been born in or about the year 1650. He matriculated at Easter, 1663, and was under the care of Dr Tenison, later Archbishop of Canterbury. He proceeded B.A. in 1666–7; M.A. in 1670; and M.D. in 1677. He was a fellow of his College 1668–82. On October 26th, 1670, he was incorporated at Oxford and then spent some time abroad at the continental schools, visiting Montpellier to work with Vieussens. Briggs was admitted a candidate of the College of Physicians in 1680 and a Fellow in 1682. In that year he gave up his fellowship at Cambridge and presumably settled in London, for he was appointed Physician to St Thomas's Hospital in the same year. He was a Censor of the College of Physicians in 1685, 1686 and 1692. He was also Physician in ordinary to King William the Third.

Dr Briggs married Hannah, daughter and heiress of Edmund Hobart, of Holt, a scion of the Hobarts of Blickling, co. Norfolk, and dying at Town Malling, in Kent, on September 4th, 1704, was buried there on September 11th. He left three children, Mary, wife of Thomas Bromfield, M.D., of London; Henry; and Hannah, wife of Dennis Martin, gent., of Loose, in Kent.† Munk gives a transcript of a long epitaph to his memory erected by his son, Henry Briggs, S.T.P., in the latter's parish church of Holt in Norfolk. This epitaph appears to have escaped the notice of Blomefield and Parkin, as they do not mention it. From it we learn that Dr Briggs was F.R.S., and that after settling in London, "he practised with great success, and soon became very eminent in his profession. He was particularly famous for his exquisite skill in difficult cases of the eye, and published two valuable treatises upon that subject".

The librarian of the Royal Society kindly informs me that although William Briggs seems to have been recognised by his contemporaries as F.R.S., there is no evidence on the records to show that he was ever proposed or regularly seconded. His

* Venn, *Alumni Cantabrigienses*, vol. I.
† Hasted, *History of Kent*, vol. II, p. 219.

name does not appear in the list of fellows, nor did he sign the charter book. There are no letters of his in the letter-books of the Society.

Munk also states that "Dr Briggs was the author of some interesting papers in the *Philosophical Transactions*, and of:

Ophthalmographia, sive Oculi ejusdem partium Descriptio Anatomica: cui accessit Nova Visionis Theoria. 12mo. Cantab. 1676.

The hypothesis of vibrations as an explanation of the phenomena of nervous action, writes Dugald Stewart, first attracted public notice in the writings of Dr William Briggs. It was from him that Sir Isaac Newton derived his anatomical knowledge; along with which he appears plainly from his *Queries* to have imbibed also some of the physiological theories of his preceptor."

Dr Briggs's portrait, by R. White, was engraved by J. Faber; this very fine mezzotint is reproduced by kind permission of the council of the Royal Society of Medicine.

This is perhaps the best place in which to correct a small slip in Garrison's *History of Medicine*, where it is stated that William Briggs described the papilla of the optic nerve in 1636. I fancy that this must be an error and that the year 1676 is meant. It is rather surprising that the *Bibliotheca Osleriana* does not appear to contain a copy of either of Dr Briggs's works. The Bowman Library possesses copies, as do the libraries of the Royal Society of Medicine, the Royal College of Surgeons and the Medical Society. They seem to have been popular in their day, for each ran through more than one edition.

OPHTHALMOGRAPHIA

This is a duodecimo in Latin of eighty pages excluding the preface, dedication and a rather full synopsis of the contents of the chapters. There are two plates of illustrations, which are crude. First published in 1676, the title-page is as follows:

Ophthalmo-graphia, | sive | Oculi ejusdem partium de- | scriptio | Anatomi-ca | Authore | Gulielmo Briggs A. M. & Coll.

PLATE IV

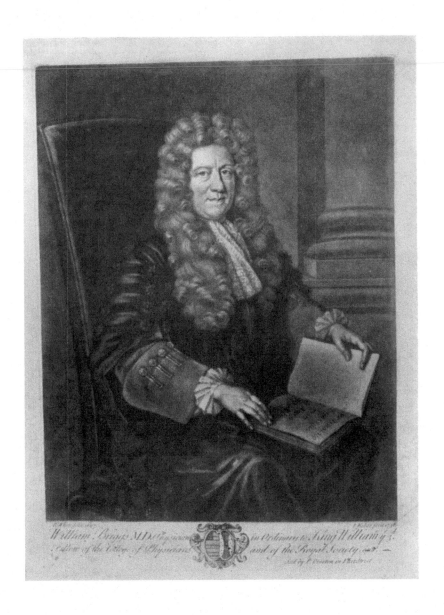

WILLIAM BRIGGS, M.D. 1650-1704

Corp. | Christi in Acad. Cantab. Socio. | Cantabrigiae, | execudebat
Joan. Hayes, Celeberrimae Academiae Ty | -pographus, impensis
Jon. Hart Bibliopolae | Cantab. 1676. |

It is dedicated to Sir Ralph Montagu, Member of the Privy
Council and late Ambassador to the King of France. Briggs
acknowledges here, and in his preface, the debt he owes to
Vieussens of Montpellier.

The second edition, also of eighty pages, was published in
1687. The title-pages of the two copies in the library of the
Royal Society of Medicine are slightly different from that of the
first edition. The first page repeats the Latin title exactly, and
goes on:

per Guilielmum Briggs, M.D. Coll. | Medic. Londin. Socium, &
Nosocomii Re- | gal. (quod Dr. Thomae dicatur) Medicum | Ordi-
narium. | Editio Secunda ab Auctore recognita. | Londini: | Typis
M.C. Impensis Ricardi Green, Bibliopolae | Cantabrigiensis,
MDCLXXXVII. |

The second title-page follows that of the first edition as far as
Socio, and then has:

Londini, | Typis M. C. Impensis Richardi Green Bibliopolae | Canta-
brigiensis. MDCLXXXVII. |

It would appear to be a reprint of the first edition and the
illustrations are the same in each.

It would be unfair to judge the anatomy in this little book by
present-day standards. The external parts together with the
muscles are fairly well described. In dealing with the obliques
Briggs cannot refrain from calling attention to their supposed
action in lovers and in the dying by interlarding a quotation from
the *Aeneid*, book 4:

> oculisque errantibus alto
> quaesivit caelo lucem ingemuitque reperta.

Dido, rolling on her couch, "and with wandering eyes she sought
the light in high heaven, and, as she found it, moaned".

Anatomists had the haziest notions as to the origin of the tunics of the eye at this date. It was generally thought that they were developed from the optic nerve and its sheaths; the nerve providing the retina and the dura and pia the sclero-cornea and choroid. In dealing with the retina Briggs specially notes and figures the papilla. But knowledge was gradually accumulating and we no longer find the lens filling the whole of the inside of the eye as in most of the earlier diagrams; and the retina is postulated as the percipient layer and not the choroid, while the function of the lens in transmitting and refracting the light is recognised. A chapter is devoted to the arteries, veins and optic nerve, in which "animal spirits" figure largely. Next follows an account of the lacrymal gland and a short chapter on peculiarities in structure of animals' eyes.

Marriotte discovered the blind spot in 1668, and as Briggs mentions his name we may conclude that his book was well up-to-date considering the age in which he lived.

Briggs was practically a contemporary of Sir Isaac Newton at Cambridge.

It is not so much on account of his *Ophthalmographia* that Briggs deserves rescuing from ophthalmic oblivion as on that of his *Nova Visionis Theoria*.

The copy of this work in the library of the Royal Society of Medicine is entitled *editio altera* and is bound up with the second edition of the *Ophthalmographia*; the *Nova Visionis Theoria* being given pride of place. It contains on the title-page the signature of "Tho. Wallis. Magd. Coll. Cant. 1718" and a note of the price paid for it, viz. 1s. 6d. Some little time ago I saw a copy for sale in a second-hand catalogue for two guineas, so that its value has appreciated.

The title-page runs as follows:

Nova Visionis | Theoria, | Regiae Societati Londin. | proposita. | per Guilielmum Briggs, M.D. Col- | leg. Medic. Londin. Socium, & | Nosocomii (quod Dr. Tho- | mae dicatur) Medicum ordinarium. | Editio Altera. | Londini: | Typis J. P. Impensis Sam. Simpson, |

Bibliopol. Cantabrig. & prostant | venales apud Sam. Smith, ad in- | signia Principis in Caemeterio D. | Pauli, Londin. 1685. |

The copy in the Bowman Library is exactly the same. The dedication to James the Second is a fulsome production, and is followed by a letter to the author from Sir Isaac Newton, and a *praeloquium* to the reader. The actual text comprises eighty duodecimo pages and there is a formidable looking illustration.

But, before discussing Briggs's New Theory, which, according to Hirschberg,* "is no theory at all though extolled by A. Hirsch", it may be of interest to record that the Bowman Library possesses another copy of both works bound together in one volume 16mo of 312 pages. This little book was published in Holland in 1686, with an engraved title-page.

This engraved page is followed by a title-page in which the titles of the two books are amalgamated as follows:

Guilielmi Briggs | Med. Doct. Colleg. Med. Londin. Soc. & | Nosocomii Regal. (quod D. Thomae dica- | tum est) Medicini Ordinarii, | OPHTHALMOGRAPHIA, | Sive | Oculi ejusdem partium | descriptio anatomica, nec non, | EJUSDEM | NOVA VISIONIS THEORIA, | Regiae Societati Londinensi | proposita. | Lugd. Batavor. | Apud PETRUM vande Aa. | MDCLXXXVI. |

This appears to be merely a reprint of the original editions, though, as there are fewer words to the line of print, the pagination is different. The illustrations are the same. It is in contemporary vellum binding and, in recording the title on the back, the binder has deprived the author of one of the "g" letters of his name; he appears as "Brigs".

Briggs's preface to the *Nova Visionis Theoria* calls attention to the fact that the *Ophthalmographia* has been already published and hints that he intends to publish later two tracts: one, *de usu partium Oculi*; the other, *de ejusdem affectibus*, if God be pleased to prolong his life.

The *Nova Visionis Theoria* was propounded before the Royal

* Hirschberg, *Geschichte der Augenheilkunde*, 2nd ed. *Graefe-Saemisch Handbuch der gesamtem Augenheilkunde*, vol. XIII, part 2, p. 319.

Society in 1681. I find that the index of the *Philosophical Transactions* lists three communications under Briggs's name. (*a*) A Discourse about vision, with an examination of some late objections, vol. XIII, p. 171. (*b*) Two remarkable cases in vision, vol. XIV, p. 559. (*c*) Philosophic solution of a case of a young man who grew blind in the evening, vol. XIV, p. 804. The first of these three contains practically the final forty-five pages of Briggs's little book, with the exception that in the *Transactions* it is given in English and in the *Nova Visionis Theoria* in Latin. He says that a specimen of his thoughts about vision appears in Mr Hook's *Philosophical Collection*, no. 6. I assume that this reference will include the first thirty-five pages of his *Theoria*.

Briggs tries to show that the fibres of the optic nerve as rising from the two protuberances of the *thalami optici* are more concerned in vision than either cornea, humours or retina (as considered by writers on optics). Sensation is performed chiefly in the brain, and these and other parts are but *transennae* to it; but also "because in Amaurosis or Gutta Serena, these parts are free from any indisposition: *i.e.*, the fibres of the optic nerve must be chiefly affected, either by obstruction by tumour, or the roots of 'em comprest about the *thalami*". He sought to prove that the superior fibres in each thalamus have the greatest tension and the inferior the least. Unless a corresponding tension exists on the two sides double vision will result. The retina examined in a glass of clear water looks like lawn or tiffany. He refers to the vibrations in a spider's web whereby impulses are conveyed from the periphery to the centre. "Rays of light strike correspondent fibres and the percussion or vibration being towards the bottom or papilla of the eye is conveyed to the nerve." "The retina is no more transparent if so much as the oil'd paper in a lantern: being white it is better able to take the images of coloured objects than the dark shade of the choroides."

Briggs's metaphor of a spider in the midst of its web, and the fibres of the retina conveying vibrations to the papilla and so to the optic thalami, is distinctly pleasing.

I think that most people will agree with Hirschberg in saying that his theory is no theory at all; but I am inclined to think that he used the Latin word *theoria* and the same word in Greek, as occurs in various parts of his thesis, to give the impression of "reflections on or thoughts concerning" vision, rather than the usual meaning of the word.

Briggs's second communication to the *Philosophical Transactions* is under date, May 20th, 1684. He gives an extract from a letter (undated) received from Dr Peter Parham, of Norwich, who reported the case of a boy, aged about 20 years, in the service of a gentleman in Suffolk, "who saw acutely and strenuously by day and was just like a post when sun set. When twilight came on he was as blind as a beetle, sees nothing, runs against gates, posts, rails (anything either higher, lower, or level to his eyes). In doors he tumbles over stools and runs his head against doors". Briggs examined the boy by daylight and in the dark and found no abnormality in the eyes. He satisfied himself that spectacles were of no use; and was inclined to attribute the lesion to the humours. He then relates another case which he saw with Dr Wm. Dawkins, at St Thomas's Hospital. It was that of a young man who was taken with dizziness and pain in the head (vertex), which he imputed to the cold weather. He went at first to a quack and was given a plaister. The pain got worse; fits made their appearance, tremor in the arms and legs and then double vision. His right eye went blind which did away with the diplopia. The treatment is outlined at some length; but the man died, and Briggs bewails the fact that he did not obtain a post-mortem examination.

The third paper is merely a short note in Latin on the case of the boy who was night-blind.

The *Nova Visionis Theoria* went out to the world with the blessing of Sir Isaac Newton, in a rather fulsome letter, in Latin, dated: Cambridge, 7, *Kal. Maii*, 1685.

Search in the Commissary Court of London and in the Prerogative Court of Canterbury has failed to discover Briggs's will. It is just possible that it may be at Canterbury. Nor was the warrant for his royal appointment discovered at the Public Record Office. The Sloane MS. 4221, fol. 189 gives a short account of Briggs which agrees closely with that in Munk's *Roll*.

Sloane MSS. 1047, 7D gives a most interesting letter addressed to Briggs. It is as follows:

Lyn, Oct. ye 26th, 1681.

Worthy Sir,

I have used Cortex Peruv. much for our agues, which have been very plentifull here. I have observed in four persons my patients, that upon taking the 2nd dose (℥ ii) they have been after 2 or 3 hours space, taken with a dimnesse, strange of sight. In a gent. aged about 46 itt took his sight away for 24 hours, and has not yett thoroughly recovered his sight, but useth spectacles to this day. In a maid servt., aged 23, itt took away her sight for three days that she could not see the way downstairs, but afterwards recovered; in a gentlewoman for severall houres, and a young gentleman the very same. I myself have been vext with an ague 14 months, and it continues still, I have taken in three quarts. of a year ℥ XIV of this cortex, itt relieved me generally for a fortnight, seldom longer, Tr. Sacra was advised by Dr Short.

Sr. I am, yr. servt.

to DR BRIGGS.   SIMON BLENCKERNE.

Sydenham is generally credited with having introduced Peruvian bark into English therapeutics for cases of ague. I am indebted to Mr Duke-Elder for the notes which follow: "the active principle of quinine was isolated in 1820 by Caventon and Peketier. Beraudi (1829) seems to have been the first to report headache, tinnitus and dimness of vision following its use. The first reported case with ophthalmoscopic examination appears to be that of von Graefe, in 1857. Both Leber and Hirschberg quote this, of von Graefe, as the first case". It is of interest to note that a general practitioner at King's Lynn anticipated the observation by more than a hundred years. In the same series of letters (Sloane MS. 1047) occurs one from John Wright, of Peterborough, dated September 25th, 1681. Addressed to Dr Briggs, it gives details of two cases, but they are of no ophthalmological interest. The first deals with the case of a marasmic baby who died convulsed during teething; the second, with the case of a man, aged about 60 years, with gonorrhoea, the details of which are not fit for publication.

The portrait of Briggs shows the family coat of arms. This is emblazoned "gules, 3 bars gemelle or, a canton argent". The sinister side of the shield contains the arms of his wife, the Hobart coat.

WILLIAM COWARD

Coward's contribution to ophthalmic literature consisted of one small volume; but he was the author of a good deal of other matter, some of it medical, but mostly metaphysical; one of the latter works was ordered to be burnt by the public hangman.

Coward was born at Winchester in 1658 and was educated at Winchester College. He was the son of William Coward of St Peter's Cheeshill, and entered college in 1668. From Winchester he went to Oxford. He matriculated at Hart Hall, in 1674, and gained a scholarship at Wadham College the next year. He graduated B.A. in 1677; fellow of Merton 1680; M.B. 1685; and M.D. 1687. He began practice at Northampton and moved to London later, settling at 93/94 Lombard Street. He was elected Candidate of the College of Physicians in 1695. It may be noted that in 1681 a Thomas Coward, possibly a relation, was Mayor of Winchester. Munk's *Roll* tells us that he came to London in 1694. Haller (*Biblioth. Med. Pract.* vol. IV, p. 177) dismisses him summarily as *non utilissimus scriptor*. He had translated into Latin, in 1682, Dryden's "Absalom and Achitophel", but this performance was surpassed by the rival translation of Atterbury. On his arrival in town he attracted considerable attention by his work entitled *Second Thoughts Concerning the Human Soul*, in which with great learning and metaphysical knowledge he united sentiments repugnant to the opinions of the best divines. This book, as well as another entitled *The Grand Essay*, in defence of it, not only drew the attacks of several writers, but the animadversions of the House of Commons, which on March 17th, 1704, ordered the latter book to be burnt by the public hangman, "as containing doctrines contrary to the Articles of the Church of England, and opposed to the Christian religion". Coward remained a Candidate of the College to the last, and died in or before 1725, having resided, it is said, for some years at Ipswich.

The title-page of his ophthalmological work is as follows:

Ophthalmiatria: | Qua Accurata & Integra | Oculorum | Male Affectorum Instituitur | Medela. | Nova Methodo Aphoristice | Concinnata. | Authore Gul. Coward, Coll. Med. Lond. M.D. | *Ars Longa, Judicium Difficile.* | Hippocrat. Aphor. I. | Impressit J. G., Impensis Joannis Chantrey e Parte | Postica Hospitii Lincolniensis; et Tho. | Atkinson ad Insigne Cygni Albi in Divi Pauli | Caemeterio, Bibliopolarum, London, 1706. |

This is a scarce little book, in octavo, of 188 pages. It is dedicated to Manuel Sorrell, a member of an old Ipswich family. The work is in Latin and hardly deserves serious consideration. He gives some formidable prescriptions for purges, and others, equally formidable, for an eye lotion. Hirschberg, in his *Geschichte*, devotes half a page to Coward. He considers him a charlatan, though he "full oft speaks of *Agyrtae*, swindlers". Hirschberg takes exception to Coward's last chapter on the proper manufacture of the *Tinctura Basilica Nostra*; but I think that Coward was quite honest in his opinions, even if mistaken. Quacks do not as a rule divulge the contents of their preparations to the world, they like to keep them secret.

Search at Somerset House failed to find Coward's will. The date of his death, 1725, is conjectural; probably he died before this and the College authorities were not informed.

ROBERT TURNER

I am indebted to Mr Arnold Sorsby for my knowledge of the little book by the above-named author. The second edition contains a section on the eye entitled "the perfect oculist" and is dated 1666. The first edition appeared without the ophthalmic appendage in 1655. The first portion, of thirty-six pages, contains the author's formularies for precious eye waters, salves, purges and clysters, etc. The second part, of twenty-eight pages, deals with certain diseases of the eye, culled chiefly from various writers. Sorsby finds that it is adapted from an anonymous tract, first published in 1616. The book is an octavo, with a frontispiece, showing, in the upper half, the portrait of the author, and below a picture of two men supporting a third, who may have dislocated his shoulder. The title-page is worth reproducing; it runs:

The Compleat | BONE SETTER | Enlarged: | Being the method of Curing | Broken Bones, dislocated Joynts, | and Ruptures, commonly called | BROKEN BELLIES. | To which is added, |

the $\begin{cases} \text{Perfect Oculist,} \\ \text{Mirrour of Health,} \\ \text{Judgment of Urines.} \end{cases}$ |

Treating of the | PESTILENCE, | And all other Diseases | written originally by Frier Moulton, Eng- | lished and Enlarged by Robert Turner Med. | The Second Edition. | London, Printed for Nath. Crouch, at the | Rose and Crown in Exchange Alley, | near Lombard-Street, 1666. |

The book is dedicated to "his honoured friend, William Chilcot jun. of Isleworth, in the County of Midd. esq." from Christopher Alley in St Martin's le Grand, June 25th, 1665. A preface to the reader ends with a puff of Turner's dentifrices, also "a soveraign antidote for the plague and all infectious diseases, foggie and unhealthy airs, Essex and Kentish agues, all of which can be bought from Mr Rooks, at the Lamb and Ink bottle, at the east end of St Paul's". But his balsam for sore eyes and for preservation of the sight could only be obtained at his own house. The main portion of the book would appear to be the work of Thomas Moulton, D.D., of the Order of the Fryers of St Augustine. This name sounds English and so this part of the book must be of a considerably earlier date than 1665. I suspect that he is the same Thomas Moulton, Dominican, calling himself Doctor of Divinity of the Order of Friars Preachers, who appears in the *Dictionary of National Biography*, and whose *Myrour or Glasse of Helthe* was published *c.* 1539. Part one of the *Perfect Oculist* takes us back to mediaeval, if not to Anglo-Saxon, ophthalmology. Fennel, rue, vervain, endive, betony, red roses, maidenhair fern, celandine, pimpernel and eyebright figure among the herbs; some solutions of metals are mentioned, and red snails, ewes' milk and woman's milk, hog's grease and the liver of a buck, without the gall, occur among the prescriptions. The powder for the eyes, called Bonaventure, was made of sugar candy and tutty, powdered and washed with rose-water, spread abroad on a basin and fumigated with lignum-aloes and frankincense, dried and powdered, to be kept in a box of brass or pewter; this powder was to be inserted with a silver pencil.

Turner's views on squint are mediaeval, and his treatment is that of "Avicen who doth commend the blood of a tuttle to be instilled; also the pye is eaten with profit, and the powder thereof is referred into a collyrium. Some suppose that the head of a Bat being burnt and powdered, others commend the head of a swallow taken by insufflation".

For "Gutta Serena, Obfuscatio, starke blindnesse or Hallucinatio" he gives a formidable prescription containing eighteen elements, to be applied to the head as a quilted cap. To strengthen weak sight the eyes of a cow are to be hung round the neck.

I am afraid that Turner must join the band of English quacks.

EARLY ROYAL OCULISTS

In January 1930 I contributed a short paper to the *British Journal of Ophthalmology* with the above title, on three men who are said to have held royal appointments: namely, Thomas Clarck, Thomas Elles (or Ellis) and Paddington Macqueen. I felt ashamed of myself at the time for the little I had been able to discover about each; and the paper was published in the hope that it might save future investigators time and trouble in knowing the search that had already been made. The illustration

PLATE V

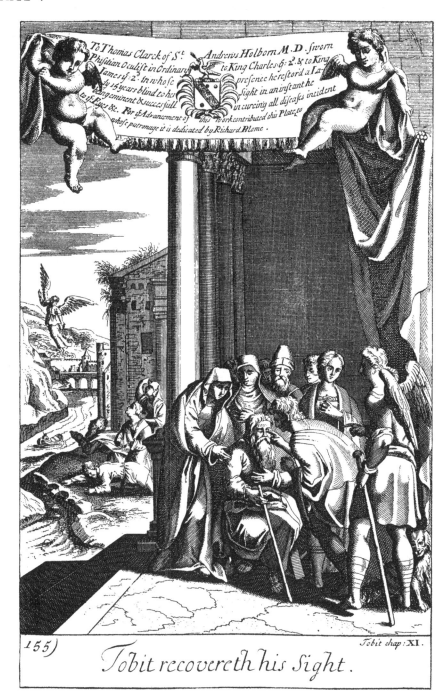

To Thomas Clark of S.t Andrew Holborn M.D. sworn Phisitian Oculist in Ordinary to King Charles 2.d & to King James 2.d In whose presence he restord a Lady 15 years blind to her sight in an instant he being eminent & successfull in cureing all diseases incident to ye Eyes &c. For ye Advancement of this Work contributed this Plate to whose patronage it is dedicated by Richard Blome.

155)

Tobit chap: XI.

Tobit recovereth his Sight.

of Tobit recovering his sight was sent to me by Mr Holmes
Spicer, to whom it had been given by Sir Anderson Critchett.
It is a rough woodcut, dedicated to Thomas Clarck, Oculist in
ordinary to Charles the Second and James the Second. It was
supposed that it might have come from a history of the Bible, by
Le Sieur de Royaumont, which was translated by J. Coughan
and J. Raynor, and printed for Robert Blome, in two volumes,
royal folio, 1690–8, with 238 plates. Mr Harvey Bloom failed
to find any trace of it at the British Museum, the British and
Foreign Bible Society and Sion College. He established the fact
that Le Sieur de Royaumont's *Histoire* does not contain the Apocrypha in either of the two editions. He was of the opinion that
this plate should have belonged to this book, but that for some
reason or other the Apocrypha was not printed. Blome did not
publish any edition of the Bible.

A Thomas Clarke, *Anglus*, figures in Peacock's *Index of
English-speaking Students who have graduated at Leyden University*,
under date March 31st, 1664. Innes Smith, in his *Students of
Medicine at Leyden*, gives this Clarke as twenty-eight years of age
and notes that he was a medical man. He surmises that possibly
the Thomas Clarke of Emmanuel College, Cambridge, 1658,
may be the same man.

In my account of Benedict Duddell (p. 96) I have mentioned
the case of a child couched for cataract by Dr Clark between the
years 1719 and 1724, and have suggested that possibly this refers
to the same man. But if the Leyden graduate was twenty-eight
years of age in 1664, he would have been born in 1636. This
would make him a very old man indeed at the date mentioned;
and although there are instances of ophthalmic surgeons continuing to practise operations up to extreme old age, I should
have thought that at the age of eighty-four or more even a quack
would have retired.

No warrant of appointment could be found at the Public
Record Office and the date of his death was not ascertained.

The *Gentleman's Magazine* for the year 1735 gave me the

following note: "Feb. 3, Thos. Elles, aet. 92, oculist to James II and Groom of the Chamber, deceased". It is of course possible that both Clarck and Elles held royal appointments at the same time, but more probable that Elles succeeded Clarck. In the *Historical Register* his name is spelt Ellis. The *Political State of England* for February 1735 says that he died at Windsor on February 27th. His body does not appear to have been buried at Windsor. Neither his will nor the record of his appointment was found.

From the same source in 1736 I obtained: "March 16, Paddington Macqueen, at Betley, Staffs., late oculist to William III, worth £16,000, deceased". The *Political State of England* for March 1736 gives: "March 9, Died at his seat in Staffordshire, Paddington Macqueen, esq. formerly oculist and groom of the Chamber to the late King".

In Macqueen's case neither will nor warrant of appointment was discovered. It is unusual to find no will in the case of one who leaves so large an estate. Macqueen was not buried at Betley.

CHAPTER VII

The Eighteenth Century

ORTHODOXY

ALTHOUGH the eighteenth century was the heyday of ophthalmic quackery, it saw the foundations laid of modern ophthalmology at the hands of those orthodox surgeons who practised in diseases of the eye in addition to general surgery. Cheselden's operation of iridotomy is a landmark in our science, and the work of Sharp and Warner in modifying the details of Daviel's operation of extraction of cataract is notable. I propose dealing with the orthodox surgeons in the first place and giving the quacks a chapter to themselves.

This century saw the rise of the voluntary hospitals, and we find that attention was being devoted to eye cases at some of the London Hospitals early in this period. Thus in 1727, John Freke was placed in charge of the eye patients at St Bartholomew's Hospital, and was authorised to couch for cataract; a fee of 6s. 8d. was paid for each couching. (Norman Moore's *History of St Bartholomew's Hospital*.) Not long afterwards, on the foundation of St George's Hospital, in 1733, we learn from Peachey's history of that institution that John Ranby, of St Thomas's Hospital and Serjeant Surgeon to George the Second, was elected to couch for cataract, although he was not formally elected a member of the staff as was his colleague, Cheselden.

On May 3rd, 1752, Handel was couched by William Bromfield, surgeon to St George's Hospital. Handel's deterioration of sight had been in evidence for about a year previously. At the close of the second act of *Jephtha*, in Handel's autograph is written the statement that "weakness of his left eye prevented him from continuing that composition". Sharp, of Guy's Hospital, was of the opinion that Handel's was a case of gutta serena. Early in 1753 it was stated in the *Theatrical Register* that "Mr Handel has quite lost his sight, although he was able to see for a little time after his operation". He appears to have been operated on thrice. The Chevalier Taylor claimed that he had operated on Handel and said he was hopeful, "but on drawing the curtain we found the bottom defective". Coats demolished this among other claims of the Chevalier (see p. 139).

PETER KENNEDY

This author's book is an octavo of 109 pages, the first 95 of which belong to the eye and the rest to diseases of the ear. There is a folding plate of illustrations. The work is entitled:

Ophthalmographia; | or, a | Treatise | of the | Eye, | in two parts. | London: | Printed for Bernard Lintott, at the Cross- | Keys between the two Temple-Gates in | Fleet Street. MDCCXIII. |

The title also contains a good deal of descriptive matter about the contents, divided into two parts, which I have not thought it worth while to abstract. Part one contains the anatomy, physiology and optics, and part two, the causes, signs and cures of maladies.

The author's name does not figure on the title-page, but he signs his dedicatory letter, which is addressed to the "learned Dr John Arbuthnot", the friend of Pope.

The contents are poor stuff, but the volume is enriched by two fine tail-pieces, one at the end of each part. In spite of the fact that the book is, ophthalmologically speaking, worthless, we must conclude that the author was an honest man. In his remarks on any condition which he considers incurable he usually ends up "as I look upon it an incurable disease, so I leave it".

WILLIAM CHESELDEN

William Cheselden was a member of the Leicestershire family of that name and was born at Somerby on October 19th, 1688. It has been stated that he began the study of his profession in his native county, but if this be true he must have started at a very tender age, for we find that, in 1703, he was a pupil of the celebrated anatomist William Cowper; and on December 7th, 1703, he was bound apprentice, for the usual term of seven years, to James Ferne, surgeon to St Thomas's Hospital. On December 5th, 1710, he was admitted to the freedom and livery of the Barber-Surgeons' Company; and he was lecturing on anatomy on his own account in 1711. Details of his career as an anatomical teacher are to be found in Peachey's *Memoir of William and John Hunter*. Peachey states that he has seen a copy of Cheselden's syllabus of anatomy in thirty-five lectures, for the use of his Anatomical Theatre, 1711; and in a footnote mentions that this is the earliest syllabus he has seen bearing the name of a private lecturer and separately printed.

In 1712 Cheselden was elected F.R.S. Two years later he was in trouble with the Barber-Surgeons' Company. In March 1714 he was admonished by the Court for contravening the by-law of the Company with regard to the procuration for the purpose of dissection of the bodies of criminals who had been executed. In 1719 he was elected surgeon to St Thomas's Hospital, with which institution he served for nineteen years; but he did not immediately relinquish his work as an anatomical teacher, for Peachey has drawn attention to an advertisement in the *Daily Courant* of March 21st, 1721, of a new course of lectures on comparative anatomy to be given by Cheselden and Francis Hawksbee. Cheselden married in 1727, and in this year was published his great surgical improvement of lateral lithotomy for vesical calculus. In 1729 he was admitted a corresponding member of the Royal Academy of Sciences of Paris, a very high honour for a surgeon; and on the formation of the Academy of Surgery of Paris, he was elected the senior foreign member of that body. In 1727 he was appointed principal surgeon to Queen Caroline, and in 1728 he gave his account of iridotomy to the world. His description is as follows: "A knife passed through the *tunica sclerotis*, under the cornea before the iris, in order to cut an artificial pupil where the natural one is clos'd. This operation I have perform'd several times with good success; indeed it cannot fail when the operation is well done, and the eye not otherwise diseas'd, which is more than can be said for couching a cataract. In this operation great care must be taken to hold open the eye lids without pressing upon the eye, for if the aqueous humour is squeez'd out before the incision is made in the iris, the eye grows flaccid and renders the operation difficult". Cheselden has also described an operation for excising a portion of a proptosed cornea, and says: "This operation is very useful, and attended with but little pain".

In 1733 Cheselden was appointed principal (consulting) surgeon to St George's Hospital, to undertake the operations for stone. He retired from St George's in 1737, when he was appointed to Chelsea Hospital. In 1743 he was chosen one of the Sheriffs of London and Middlesex, but he swore off. Two years later, when he was junior warden of the Barber-Surgeons' Company, the separation of the surgeons and the barbers took place. He was elected one of the wardens of the Company of Surgeons on its foundation, and in the following year, Master. Wadd relates that Cheselden was a patron of the arts, and states that the plan of Fulham Bridge was drawn by him. He was a patron of boxing and sports generally; his disposition was gay and genial, and he had the reputation of being kind to his patients. His portrait is the most striking of those which adorn the walls of the Council Room at the Royal College of Surgeons. Cheselden had an apoplectic stroke in 1751 and died at Bath on April 10th, 1752. His will is one of the briefest on record.

To the general public Cheselden is probably best known through the reference to him by Pope. The poet had been under Cheselden's care in 1736, possibly for a complaint in his eyes. The couplet is as follows:

> Weak tho' I am of limb, and short of sight,
> Far from a lynx and not a giant quite,
> I'll do what MEAD and CHESELDEN advise,
> To keep these limbs, and to preserve these eyes.

The following letter from Pope to Cheselden is printed in Roscoe's life of Pope (1824):

Dear Sir,

You know my laconic style. I never forget you. Are you well? I am so. How does Mrs Cheselden? Had it not been for her, you had been here. Here are three cataracts ripened for you (Mr Pierce assures me). Adieu. I do not intend to go to London. Good night, but answer me.   yours, A. POPE.

Bath, Nov. 21.

P.S. Shew this to Mr Richardson, and let him take it to himself, and to his son. He has no wife.

To Mr Cheselden.

BENEDICT DUDDELL

Coats, in his memoir of the Chevalier Taylor (*Moorfields Hospital Reports*, vol. xx, p. 22), says that Duddell was "the best English writer on ophthalmic subjects in the first half of the eighteenth century"; and Hirschberg (in *Graefe-Saemisch*, vol. XIII, p. 125) devotes more than six pages to him. I have found him an elusive personage. He says in the preface to his first publication (*vide infra*), that his reason for taking up the study of diseases of the eye was "the misfortune of a poor man at Worksop, Nottinghamshire; who, notwithstanding my best endeavours, lost his sight; and in consequence the means of providing for a numerous family of starving children". He must have been in practice at Worksop at this time. He goes on to say that in 1718 he went to Paris to study under a very eminent oculist, whom Hirschberg identifies as Woolhouse. He notes also that formerly he had served his apprenticeship but four leagues from Paris.

His first book is an octavo of 232 pages, published in 1729 with the following title:

A | Treatise | of the | Diseases | of the | Horny-Coat of the Eye, | and the | various kinds of Cataracts. | To which is prefix'd, | A Method, entirely new, of scarifying | the Eyes for several Disorders.

| with remarks on the practice of some | Oculists both at home and Abroad. | by Benedict Duddell, | Surgeon and Oculist. | London: | Printed for John Clark at the Royal Ex- | change, and sold by J. Roberts in Warwick- | Lane. MDCCXXIX. |

His main reason for writing this book was to correct certain errors in the Chevalier Taylor's *Mechanism of the Eye*. Coats says "his tone is critical, but not hostile; he disagrees with Taylor's method of treating corneal nebulae and with his classification of opacities of the lens, draws attention to the importance of observing the mobility of the pupil before operating for cataract, and answers certain queries which Taylor had propounded". In a later work "he gives an unfavourable account of the Chevalier's operating, saying that his hand shook, that vitreous was lost, and that his method of performing the operation for cataract did not correspond with his descriptions".

In his preface he condemns those surgeons who attempt to treat eye cases without having made a special study of such conditions. The following sentence may be quoted in this respect: "to the question how a certain surgeon did to know the different natures of the distempers of the eye: His answer was that he undertook all. If his operation succeeded, so much the better; if not, the patients cou'd but be blind, or in danger of being so, as they were before".

His first chapter contains a good account of the anatomy of the parts. His second deals with distempers of the Horny-Coat. The place of honour is given to a description of his new scarifyer, which is as follows: "Take about 25 beards of barley, placing the upper ends downwards; break them off about 3 quarters of an inch long; tye them from the middle down to your fingers, and this makes a little brush". It was found in practice that sometimes little bits of barley beard broke off and remained in the conjunctival sac; and, in a later book, he advises that the brush be made from the beards of wheat, as being stronger. This apparatus seems to have been his chief instrument in most of the disorders of the eye save where couching was indicated. He scarified the conjunctiva of the lids and globe but took care to avoid touching the cornea. Warm water bathing, with brandy added occasionally, and a poultice at night, made from the pulp of a roasted apple, formed the major part of the rest of his local treatment. For general treatment he indulged in low diet, resting flat in bed, bleeding and purgation, with mercury in selected cases.

He relates many interesting cases: one, of albugo, due to a lime burn, with partial symblepharon, was treated by division of the latter, scarification and oily applications, with some improvement.

He frequently refers to the works of Woolhouse and St Yves, occasionally to Banister and once to Benevenutus Grassus, whose name he mis-spells. A case of perforating wound of the eye is recounted: "A busy old woman had applied a plaister", and the boy was in much pain. His treatment was rest, flat in bed, with low diet for fear of inflammation with the inevitable scarification, especially when the eye was painful. The pain in this case was ascribed to "the uvea digested came through the wound in the cornea". Five weeks later the eye was soundly healed. "The eye that is not hurt must always be drest for fear of a flux of humours upon it: I have seen several that have lost both eyes, though only one has been hurt at first, by reason of bad applications, and irregular methods." Here we have an early suspicion of sympathetic ophthalmitis.

"The reputation of the surgeon and the loss of the patient's sight very often go together" is an observation which contains a great truth. Ingrowing lashes Duddell calls *phalangosis*. Many of his cases appear to have been seen in Hammersmith; he went as far as Richmond, in Surrey, to Acton and White-Chapel.

Ragoides would appear to be a large prolapse of iris; he recommends tying it off with a ligature; a bigger prolapse involves the choroid and is called *melon*.

"The eyes of persons turned of sixty should be scarified every three months to maintain the fluidity of the juices and prevent opacity." There is a long chapter on lacrymal fistulae and their treatment; and the rest of the book deals with cataract. He gives a good account of such early symptoms as motes, polyopia, cobweb, etc.; and is insistent that softness of the globe is a bad sign in cataract. So far as I observed he does not make any mention of hardness of the eye in glaucoma. In order to detect a gutta serena complicating a cataract, the method of Peter Kennedy, transcribed by Arnold Sorsby, in his article on Banister in the *British Journal of Ophthalmology* (May 1932), is given almost word for word.

"In couching the operator must pass his needle 2 or 3 times through the lap of his coat, to warm the needle, because it being cold, it will be subject to stop the pores, and occasion an inflammation." German and Northern oculists use a round needle which "they moisten with their spittle". According to the late Johnson Taylor, of Norwich, Bell Taylor, of Nottingham, used to spit on his knife before putting it away.* Many cataract cases are recorded; one, a child, had been given up as hopeless by Sir William Reed (*sic*); Duddell made a hole in a shrunken membrane and improved the sight. Another of his cases, a child, had been couched by Dr Clark between 1719 and 1726; possibly this may have been the John Clark, Oculist to James the Second (*q.v.*).

Duddell advised the forerunner of a cartella shield, by boring a hole in half a walnut shell, blackening the inside, and tying it over the operated eye. He uses the word hippus to denote nystagmus.

In 1733 he brought out a second volume, also in octavo, of 136 pages. This is entitled:

An | Appendix | to the | Treatise | of the | Horny-Coat of the Eye, | and the Cataract. | with an | Answer | to Mr. Cheselden's Appendix, re- | lating to his new operation | upon the iris of the Eye. | by Benedict Duddell. Surgeon. | London: | Printed by E. Howlatt, and sold at the Gol- | den-Ball in Bullin-Court, near the New | Exchange in the Strand. Price two | shillings stitched. 1733. |

* *British Journal of Ophthalmology*, vol. VI, p. 93.

In the preface he draws attention to Taylor's errors in the *Mechanism of the Eye*, "notably in the matter of pareing the cornea for a cartilaginous excrescence of that coat". The main part of the book consists of case reports. One of Cheselden's cases of iridotomy, which had become blind, is described and criticised. He then wanders off into venereal complaints, cases of retention of urine and other non-ophthalmic matters, and ends with an account of the eye of the horse.

His third book, of sixty-one pages, is entitled:

A | Supplement | to the | Treatise | of the | Diseases of the Horny-Coat and | Cataract of the Eye, and its | Appendix. | by Benedict Duddell. Surgeon. London: | Printed for J. Roberts, near the Oxford- | Arms in Warwick-Lane 1736. |

In the preface he has a dig at Taylor's mountebank performances at "his house in Suffolk Street, the 16th of August last, where eyes were turned inside out, and vision tossed about; which operations were inconsistent with the rules of surgery".

I have been unable to find out the date of Duddell's death, and search at Somerset House has failed to find his will. There are no letters of his at the British Museum.

SHARP & WARNER

To appreciate the contributions of these two distinguished surgeons of Guy's Hospital, it is necessary to allude to the extraction operation for cataract propounded by Daviel in 1752. Before that date couching had been the only treatment for cataract from time immemorial. Daviel's operation was clumsy, in that he made a puncture incision at the limbus below and enlarged it on each side with scissors. Samuel Sharp invented a rather beak-shaped knife in order to make the incision from within outwards after puncture and counter-puncture; his knife is the forerunner of the more perfect linear knife of von Graefe.

Samuel Sharp was born about 1700 and was a pupil of Cheselden at St Thomas's Hospital. He also studied at Paris and in 1733 was elected surgeon to Guy's Hospital. Early in his career he was lecturing on anatomy and surgery to the Society of Naval Surgeons; this office he resigned in favour of William Hunter in 1747. Ten years later ill-health compelled him to resign his post at Guy's. In 1750 he published his *Critical Inquiry into the Present State of Surgery*. In 1753 appeared in the *Philosophical Transactions* his "New Method of Opening the Cornea in order to extract the Crystalline Humour". Sharp was a F.R.S. and in 1749 was elected a member of the French Academy of Surgery. In the winter of 1765–6 he made a continental tour, visiting France and Italy. His *Letters from Italy* appeared in August 1766 and was promptly answered by Sam. Johnson's friend, Baretti, who thought that aspersions had been cast upon his native country.

In the operation of iridotomy Sharp introduced a long straight knife with a slightly concave cutting edge between the ciliary ligament and the iris; made it penetrate the anterior chamber of the eye, with the back of the knife turned towards the cornea, and when the point reached the side opposite to its entrance, he incised the membrane, and at the same time withdrew the knife.

Daviel recommended opening the capsule of the lens in his operation of extraction of cataract. Sharp thought this dangerous and unnecessary. Sometimes, he says, after the section is completed, the aqueous, lens and vitreous "fly out". If this should happen he advises that the eye be tied up quickly. If the lens does not come out easily, pressure on the lower part of the cornea should be made; the cataract should then advance through the pupil into the anterior chamber, whence it will pass through the wound. If the lens does not readily present, its exit can be assisted by lifting it from its bed by the knife previously stuck into it. This is likely to avoid the danger of "evacuating the whole or too much of the vitreous which is apt to follow the cataract when the eye is firmly pressed".

In spite of his ill-health Sharp lived until March 24th, 1778. This account of him is largely drawn from Wilks and Bettany's *History of Guy's Hospital*. From the same source the biographical facts which follow about Joseph Warner are mainly drawn.

The will of a certain Samuel Sharpe (P.C.C., Hay, 172) was signed on November 20th, 1775 and proved on May 4th, 1778. I do not feel sure that this is the will of the surgeon as it contains no evidence to that effect. After mentioning various small legacies he leaves his "daughter Elenor 45s. yearly, my house in the Circuss and £6070; and to daughter Frances her annuity of 28s. and £7870. The furniture of his house in the Circuss, which was left to daughter Elenor, to be divided among his three daughters; his books among his four children, and the remainder of the estate to son Samuel Pocklington. His brother-in-law, Daniel Bayne, was to have his gold watch and to be executor with daughter Elenor. The witnesses are Wm. Buckle, Wm. Nassau Elliott and G. Rooper". There are no fewer than eight codicils.

Joseph Warner was born in Antigua in 1717; he was educated at Westminster and apprenticed to Sharp at the age of seventeen. He volunteered for active service in the '45 and was in Scotland. A surgeon of the name of Cowell was also present with the forces; both Warner and Cowell were contemplating applying for the post of surgeon to St Thomas's Hospital. The vacancy was declared while they were in Scotland and Cowell got to know about it. Without mentioning the matter to Warner he obtained leave of absence on account of urgent business in London. Cowell was elected and it is stated that Warner never forgave him this piece of sharp practice. Wadd (*Mems., Maxims, and Memoirs*) tells the story that whenever afterwards Warner met his colleagues at the Court of Assistants at Surgeons' Hall, he invariably accosted them thus: "How d'ye do, gentlemen? I am glad to see you all, except Mr Cowell".

A letter from Warner, addressed to John Gunning, of St George's Hospital, under date December 29th, 1792, deals with the arrangements at the Borough hospitals for teaching and is of interest in connexion with the squabble which caused the death of John Hunter. Warner was elected surgeon to Guy's Hospital very soon after his return from Scotland. In 1754 he published *Cases in Surgery*. He also published a *Description of the Human Eye, with its Diseases*; this appeared in 1773 and a second edition was brought out in 1775. He is reputed to have been a good operator in eye cases. He died in 1801.

The following account of Warner's operation for extraction of cataract is taken from Chandler's *Treatise on the Diseases of the Eye*, 1780.

The manner in which this operation (Warner's) may be performed is as follows: The patient being seated upon a large trunk, or box, the operator places himself exactly opposite, upon a seat of a convenient height, and in a room where the light is moderate, that the pupil may not be too much contracted.

This being done an assistant stands behind the patient, who puts his right hand under the patient's chin, after having covered the right eye, supposing it to be the left which is to be operated upon: the assistant then places the back part of the patient's head on his breast, at the same time directing the face upwards, to prevent the sudden discharge of the vitreous humor. He afterwards lifts up the superior eyelid with two or more of his fingers, taking care not to press upon the globe of the eye above: the operator at the same time depresses the inferior eyelid, with this precaution, not to press upon the inferior part of the globe of the eye till the incision is made. The patient must look straight forwards, and a little upwards. The operator now fixes his right elbow upon his right knee; after having put his right foot firmly on the patient's seat for this purpose. He then suddenly and resolutely introduces the point of his knife through the external part of the cornea, opposite to the centre of the pupil, directing it horizontally betwixt the anterior surface of the iris, and the interior surface of the cornea, into the fore-chamber of the eye, till it penetrates through the cornea on its opposite side; when the inferior part of the cornea must be suddenly divided, by directing the blade of the knife downwards and outwards. The larger and lower the incision is made the better will the operation be likely to succeed; and if it happens that the wound thro' the cornea proves too small it must be enlarged by a pair of sharp scissars, well polished; the blade of which must be curved so that they may have a convex and concave surface.

The next process of the operation is to wound the aranea. This ought not to be attempted till a few minutes after the cornea has been incised: as soon as the incision is made through the cornea the eyelids should be set loose. By paying a proper attention to these maxims the whole of the aqueous humor will be evacuated; the iris will

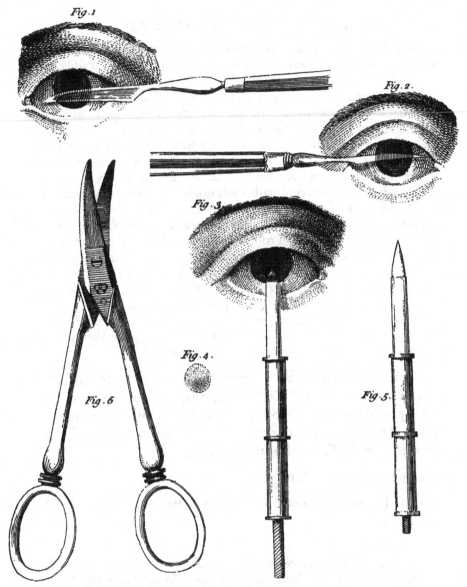

Fig. 1. The eye with Mr Warner's knife passing thro' the cornea.

Fig. 2. Mr Sharp's knife *in situ*.

Fig. 3. The eye with the wound on the inferior part of the cornea, with the instrument passed under the cornea and lying upon the iris, for dividing the aranea.

Fig. 4. The cataract.

Fig. 5. The instrument for dividing the aranea with the point of the lancet out of its case.

Fig. 6. The curved scissars for enlarging the wound of the cornea.

become flaccid and subside upon the cataract: the pupil will be dilated, and the instrument for cutting thro' the capsula may then readily be directed under the flap of the cornea to the inferior edge of the pupil. From these precautions the pupil will escape violence: to which it is very liable from the passage of the cataract through it when contracted and small. Immediately after the membrane is wounded the globe of the eye must be pressed gently upwards, that the cataract may be squeezed thro' the pupil and inferior part of the cornea, where the incision has been made. The cataract being thus removed the eyelids must be covered with a soft double or triple rag, dipped in a cold solution of saccharum saturni, or the pulvis cerussa comp. prepared in damask rose water, or spring water: this application must be kept on with a soft linen roller, and renewed two or three times a day. The patient must be laid on his back upon a bed or couch; and in this situation he must keep himself for some days that the wound made through the cornea may heal, and the newly secreted aqueous humor may be prevented from escaping out of the eye.

During the inflammatory state the eye should be treated with emollient fomentations and the patient's body must be kept open: opiates likewise must occasionally be administered.

There are no letters by Warner in the British Museum. The librarian of the Royal College of Surgeons of England has kindly given me permission to transcribe for publication in this book the following letter from the "Stone Collection", the property of the Council of the College.

Stone Collection, vol. III, p. 92.

To the Master: Wardens; & Court of Assistants of the Surgs. Company

Gentlemen—

With all due respect & Deference to this Court, I take the liberty of offering the following opinion: To wit, that the Surgs. Company does not, has not, & probably can not sustain any loss; or experience any obstruction; or the least degree of inconvenience, from the Building, which is now erecting, by the City of London, above that Footpassage, to the whole, or at least one half of which the Surgeon's Company do claim an indisputable right: for the above stated reasons, I can not think, that we ought to proceed with any degree of precipitation, or violence upon this occasion: & more especially so, as the City of London may possibly be possessed of some reason, or reasons, for what it is now doing (besides that important Plea of public Good) with which reason, or reasons, we at present are quite unacquainted.

Should these few suggestions, to this Court appear to be not of the least weight, I am nevertheless induced to conjecture, that the most adviseable Part for us to take is to proceed in a temperate; regular; & circumspect manner upon this question: as well as upon every other matter, that concerns the Surgeons Company at large: as well as our own Characters, as (*being the) Court of Assistants (*& Guardians) of that Company; for the honor, & benefit of which, We have been summoned to convene on this Day.

I am very respectfully
Gentlemen,
your most obed^t. & ·
very humble servant
JOSEPH WARNER.

Hatton Garden.
Sept. 19, 1792.

Warner's will (P.C.C., Abercrombie, 562) is dated November 17th, 1800, and was proved on August 4th, 1801. In it he describes himself as surgeon, of Hatton Street, St Andrew's, Holborn. He desires to be buried without show and with as much economy as possible in the New Burying Ground belonging to St Andrew's in Gray's Inn Lane near the body of his daughter, Mary Warner. The bulk of his property he left to his wife, Elizabeth, including his dwelling-house in Hatton Street. After her death the house was to go to his son Joseph Warner. Bequests to various grandsons and to his daughter, Elizabeth Thornton, are detailed. Son Joseph to have £50 for mourning and the same sum is left to his daughter-in-law, Mildred Warner. To his grandson Joseph Thomas Warner £100, "who after my decease will represent the eldest branch of the family, Queen Elizabeth's diamond ring, which has long and regularly descended in the family as an heirloom". After bequests to his

* Insertions.

housekeeper and maidservants the will ends: "Half estate to son Joseph, the other to son Joseph and grandson Joseph Thomas, in trust to pay daughter Elizabeth Thornton to her own use in spite of Robert Thornton her present husband". His son Joseph is named executor. The will is witnessed by Ashley Balfour and William Shaw.

JAMES WARE

An account of James Ware was contributed to the first volume of the *British Journal of Ophthalmology* by the late Percy Dunn; but most of the facts recorded here are from the life of Ware in Pettigrew's *Medical Portrait Gallery*.

James Ware was the son of a master shipbuilder of Deptford and was born at Portsmouth in 1756. He was educated at the Portsmouth Grammar School and apprenticed to Mr Ramsay Karr, surgeon, of Portsmouth. Later he entered the school of St Thomas's Hospital. He learnt his ophthalmology from Wathen (*q.v.*) and went into partnership with him for fourteen years. The partnership was dissolved in 1791 and he began practice on his own account. Ware was a prolific author.

In 1780 he published *Remarks on the Ophthalmy, Psorophthalmy and Purulent Eye*. A second edition of this book appeared in 1787 and a third in 1795; while it was republished in 1805 in his *Chirurgical Observations relative to the Eye*. He gave the name psorophthalmy to cases of inflammation with ulceration of the lids and showed its frequent connexion with a scrofulous diathesis. For the purulent eyes of new-born children he relied chiefly on the *Aqua Camphorata* of Bate's Dispensatory. Appended to this work is the account of a case of gutta serena cured by electricity.

In 1791 appeared Ware's translation of Baron de Wenzel's treatise on cataract. In the following year he brought out his *Chirurgical Observations relative to the Epiphora, or Watery Eye; the Scrophulous and Intermittent Ophthalmy; the Extraction of*

PLATE VI

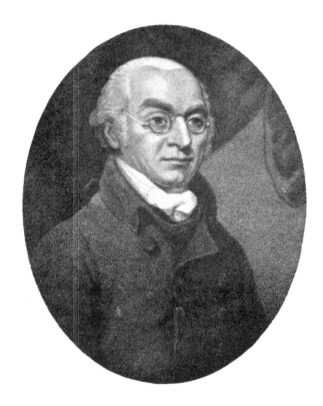

JAMES WARE

Cataract; and the Introduction of the Male Catheter. He seems to have followed the method of Anel in treating lacrymal obstruction; the cases of intermittent ophthalmy seem to have been of a syphilitic nature as they yielded to mercury; while the scrofulous variety benefited by Peruvian bark, conjoined with soda.

In 1795 he published

An Enquiry into the Causes which have most commonly prevented success in the Operation of Cataract; with an account of the means by which they may be either avoided or rectified. To which are added, Observations on the Dissipation of the Cataract, and on the cure of Gutta Serena. Also additional Reflections on the Epiphora, or Watery Eye.

Ware condemns the practice of publishing only cases of success in treatment, without fairly stating the disadvantages or accidents to which it is liable. With regard to the accidents which may occur in the extraction of cataract, his opinion is that these mainly result from (1) too small a corneal incision; (2) wounding the iris; (3) loss of vitreous; (4) incomplete extraction, part of the lens being left in the eye; (5) undue pressure after the operation; (6) exposure of the eyes prematurely to too strong light.

Some cases of gutta serena, cured by electricity, and other cases, cured by mercurial snuff, are included in this book.

In 1798 appeared his *Remarks on Fistula Lachrymalis; with the Description of an Operation considerably different from that commonly used; to which are added, Observations on Haemorrhoids, and additional Remarks on the Ophthalmy.* Ware proposed the introduction of a style in cases of lacrymal obstruction, and his operation is illustrated by a plate. Pott and Warner had treated such cases by opening the sac, dilating it with a sponge tent, passing a piece of catgut or puncturing the os unguis. Previously to this date Wathen had attempted the passage of a canula. The additional remarks on ophthalmy resolve themselves into emphasising the value of the Thebaic tincture, of the London Pharmacopoeia, 1745, and not the ordinary tincture of opium of the "present" edition.

The *Chirurgical Observations on the Eye*, with an Appendix, appeared in 1805, in two volumes; the first consists mainly of reprints of his previous shorter works, while the second contains his translation of de Wenzel's treatise on cataract, together with his own remarks on this subject. This volume contains his account of the cure of a boy who recovered his sight at the age of seven years, after having been deprived of it by cataracts before he was a year old. This case was communicated to the Royal Society, of which Ware was a fellow, in 1801 and was printed in the *Philosophical Transactions*.

In 1808 appeared his *Remarks on the Prevalent Ophthalmy, which has lately been epidemical in this Country*. This ophthalmia seems to have been partly gonorrhoeal conjunctivitis and partly trachoma. To the *Memoirs of the Medical Society of London* Ware contributed three papers; the first on a case of retention of urine, the second on a successful cataract case of long standing, and the third, his cases of gutta serena, cured by electricity. He also contributed to vol. 1 a paper on staphyloma, hydrophthalmia and carcinoma of the eye.

The *Transactions of the Medico-Chirurgical Society* contain a paper by him on muscae volitantes of nervous persons. Besides the paper in the *Philosophical Transactions* already mentioned he contributed one, read in November 1812, on the near and distant sight of different persons.

In 1818 his son, Martin Ware, reprinted some of his father's tracts in order to complete the collection of his works.

Ware was a philanthropist. He was one of the founders of the School for the Indigent Blind, in 1800; and he was a founder of the Society for the Relief of the Widows and Orphans of Medical Men in London and its Vicinity. In 1809 he was elected president of this society, a society which still continues to exist in a flourishing condition. Ware married in 1787 the widow of N. Polhill, Esq., who was the daughter of an opulent city merchant, Robert Maitland; they had a large family. He died in April, 1815.

In a copy of Scarpa's *Diseases of the Eye*, in my possession, is written the following doggerel verse:

> Your eyes are so bad, you'd do well to repair
> And seek the assistance of oculist Ware.
> Not I, by my faith, for so bad as they are,
> Is mainly, nay solely, occasioned by Wear.

Abstract of will of JAMES WARE (P.C.C., Pakenham, 216).

JAMES WARE, of New Bridge Street, London.
Dated June 6th, 1812.

To wife Ursula £10,000 3 % Consolidated Bank annuities, household goods, plate, jewels, prints and pictures.

To son-in-law Robert Joseph Chambers of Beech Hill, Waltham Abbey, esq. £1,000.

Executors to buy £24,000 3 % Consolidated Bank securities for my children. Freeholds in Aylesbury, bought of Sir John Packington Bart. and freehold in Chancery Lane bought of the exors. of John Gorham, esq. to wife for life, and on her death the Aylesbury estate to son Martin and another part to my daughter Ursula Ware and my son James Ware; and that part occupied by Joseph Watkins to my sons Robert Ware and Ebenezer Ware. Son Martin may purchase my house in New Bridge St. Houses in William St. and King Edward St. for £2,000 to the use of my wife and her brothers John and Alexander Maitland. Copyholds at Turnham Green, held of the Manor of Sutton Court and freehold rents in Bear binder Lane, Swithin's Lane and Dove Court, bought of Sir John Frederick, and a mess. on west of Abchurch Lane, bought of the Earl of Lauderdale and now in the tenure of the Postmaster General and my freeholds in Peter St. and Green's Court, Westminster and freehold house in Colebrook Row, Islington; leaseholds in New Bridge St. and William St. to the use of my wife and her said brothers as trustees. To sister Mary Godwin 30 guineas and to my sisters Elizabeth Ware and Ann Harriss £200 3 % annuities. To the treasurer of the Socy for the relief of Widows and Orphans of medical men in London £200 3 % annuities. To the School for the Indigent Blind, established in London, 1799, £100.

There are bequests of £20 to two servants; and rings are stipulated to be given to nephew and niece Kelly, Mrs Whitaker, Mrs Bliss, and Mrs Barnes. The residue in trust: to pay wife interest for life to daughter-in-law Elizabeth Polhill and her children. His wife and her two brothers to be executors. There is a codicil of no interest. Proved April 29th, 1815, by Ursula and John and Alexander Maitland and Martin and James Ware, his sons.

THOMAS GATAKER

I published a short account of Gataker in the *Archives of Ophthalmology* in February 1932. His contribution to the ophthalmic science of his day was meagre, consisting of a small volume, of eighty-six pages octavo, published in 1761. This little book consists of a series of three lectures on the anatomy of the eye, which were given in the theatre of Surgeons' Hall. In some ways it marks a turning-point between old and new views. Thus, Gataker is sceptical as to the old notion that the three coats of the eye were derived from the optic nerve and its sheaths, but thinks that it may be "proper to retain the old opinion till a more certain one is established". He mentions that fleshy fibres have been described between the duplicatures of the ciliary body, and says that modern enquiries do not confirm their existence. "There is reason to believe that, by their numerous villi, the ciliary processes contribute very considerably to the secretion of the aqueous humour. One opinion of their use has been more generally received, namely, that by their contraction, the crystalline and vitreous are brought forward, making the cornea more prominent, as when we would view small and near objects distinctly; but as the existence of muscular fibres in the ciliary processes is by no means proved, it may be reasonably doubted whether the actions of these processes can have any power in the motion of these humours."

The aqueous humour, he says, is secreted from the blood, and being formed constantly, there must be some arrangement whereby the excess is removed. How this is done is not clearly established, but "it is probable that part is taken up by the absorbent veins and part of it may transpire through the cornea". In some of this Gataker seems to have been within measurable distance of present-day views.

Gataker was descended from the ancient Shropshire family of Gatacre of Gatacre. His father was the Rev. Edward Gataker, Rector of Mursley, Bucks. The date of Thomas Gataker's birth has not been ascertained; he was apprenticed at Barber-Surgeons' Hall on December 2nd, 1731, to Isaac Rider, Surgeon, of London, for the usual period of seven years. Eleven years later he was admitted to the freedom of the Company, "by servitude". In 1754 he was elected surgeon to the Westminster Hospital and in 1760 to St George's Hospital. He died in 1768 and was succeeded at St George's by John Hunter.

Gataker was the author of several small books on general medical topics, and refers in one of his prefaces to a work on cataract which apparently was not published. I am under the impression that he intended to contrast the results obtained in cataract cases by the old couching operation with those resulting from extraction; but he seems to have thought that the time was not then ripe for an authoritative pronouncement on this question. His largest work was his translation, from the French, of Le Dran's *Operations of Surgery*. His widow and two children survived him. His will (P.C.C., Secker, 412) was proved in London by his widow on November 28th, 1768; it was dated September 29th, 1768, and is a short document of no particular interest; among the witnesses is William Walker, his apprentice, who was one of Hunter's opponents at St George's. The fact that Gataker was a regular attendant at Board meetings at the hospital until June 3rd, 1768, makes it clear that his last illness was of short duration.

WILLIAM CHARLES WELLS, M.D., F.R.S.

Wells's chief contribution to ophthalmology was his essay on single vision with the two eyes. I contributed a paper on him to the *British Journal of Ophthalmology* in November 1928, founded upon the autobiography included in his collected works (1818).

He was the son of Scottish parents and was born in South Carolina in May 1757. His father had emigrated from Dundee to America, in 1753, to engage in mercantile business; this failing, he set up as a bookbinder and bookseller. His son was sent home at eleven years of age to attend the Dumfries School. In 1770 he attended the lower classes in the University of Edinburgh, and returning to Carolina in the next year, he was apprenticed to Dr Alexander Garden, at that time the chief physician in Charlestown. Wells's manners, "rude and rough from his infancy", had been polished at Edinburgh, where he had as friends David Hume and William Miller, afterwards Lord Glenlee; but he got on badly with Dr Garden and his fellow pupils, most of whom were of low standard. Before his indentures were completed the rebellion broke out in New England and the Wells family returned to England. The younger Wells went to Edinburgh, but did not graduate then. He entered at St Bartholomew's Hospital and then became surgeon to a Scottish regiment in Holland. He joined his regiment in 1779. His colonel bore the good Scots name of Hamilton, but could hardly speak English and the two were quickly at daggers drawn; Wells resigned his commission and early in 1780 spent three months at Leyden, occupying himself with a thesis (*de Frigore*) on which he graduated at Edinburgh later in the year. For the next three years he was in Carolina trying to clear up his father's affairs, and after experiencing much hardship, he left America in 1784 and came to London. Here he gained the friendship of Matthew Baillie, to whom the collected edition of his works is dedicated. Most of Wells's after-career in town was passed in penury. He was elected physician to the Finsbury Dispensary in 1790, and, five years later, to St Thomas's Hospital. In 1793 he was elected F.R.S. and later the Society awarded him the Romford medal for his essay on dew. His essay on vision was published in 1792. In 1800 he had an apoplectic fit and in consequence gave up much of his work, confining himself to literary pursuits. He died on September 18th, 1817, and was buried at St Bride's, Fleet Street.

His essay is divided into three parts: the first of which is a criticism of the views of previous authors, from Galen to

Porterfield; the second part deals with Wells's own theory respecting visible direction; while the third part amplifies the foregoing section and offers an explanation of some other phenomena of vision.

It must be confessed that Wells's essay makes rather dull reading; I dealt fully with it in my previous paper and here offer merely an abstract of part of it.

The second part of his essay is Wells's own theory respecting visible direction, and his solution hence derived of the question, why objects are seen single with the two eyes. The following explanation of terms is offered.

(1) When a small object is so placed with respect to either eye, as to be seen more distinctly than in any other situation, I say it is then in the optic axis, or the axis of that eye; and if another small body be interposed between the former and the eye, so as to conceal it, and if a line joining the two be produced till it falls upon the cornea, I call this line the *optic axis*, or the axis of the eye; leaving for future determination the precise point of the cornea it falls upon or what part of the retina receives the picture of an object which is placed in it. (2) When the two optic axes are directed to a small object not very distant, they may be conceived to form two sides of a triangle, the base of which is the interval between the points of the corneas where the axes enter the eyes; but if the object be very distant, then they may be supposed to be two sides of a parallelogram whose base is the same interval. To avoid circumlocution I shall call this interval the *visual base*. (3) If there be a line drawn from the middle of the visual base through the point of intersection of the optic axes, or parallel to them, if they be parallel to each other, I name it the *common axis*. The term I believe was invented by Alhazen, but with him it signified a line drawn from the centre of the junction of the optic nerves, through the middle of the interval between the centres of the retinas. Such a line was consequently immovable. As the term, however, is not in modern use, no mistake can arise from confounding the two meanings, and the reason will soon be seen why I employ it in the sense I have mentioned. Those who are acquainted with the writings of the older opticians, will perceive that I give it nearly the same signification as they did to their *common radius*.

Wells next proceeds to prove the following propositions:

(1) Objects, situated in the optic axis, do not appear to be in that line, but in the common axis. (2) Objects, situated in the common axis, do not appear to be in that line, but in the axis of the eye, by which they are seen. (3) Objects, situated in any line drawn through the mutual intersection of the optic axes to the visual base, do not appear to be in that line, but in another drawn through the same intersection to a point in the visual base distant half this base from the similar extremity of the former line, towards the left, if the objects be seen by the right eye, but towards the right, if seen by the left eye.

JONATHAN WATHEN

Besides some tracts on general surgical matters, Wathen published two small pamphlets on ophthalmic subjects. The first of these seems to have run into two editions, the second of which is entitled:

A New and Easy | Method of Curing | the | Fistula Lacrymalis: | The second edition, with considerable improvements. | To which is added | A Dissertation | on the | Epiphora Vera; | or, True Watery Eye: | and the | Zerophthalmia; | or, Dry Eye. | by Jonathan Wathen, Surgeon. F.A.S. | Also, | An Appendix, | on the Treatment of Patients after the | Operation for the Cataract: | in which are shewn, | The evils attendant on long confinement and continued | Bandages; and an opposite Practice recommended. | Illustrated with Cases. | by Jonathan Wathen Phipps,* Surgeon. | London: | Printed for C. Dilly, in the Poultry. | 1792. |

This tract, in spite of its overloaded title, is a short one; it is dedicated from Pall Mall, July 1st, 1792, to John Hunter. It appears that the first edition, which I have not seen, was published in 1781. Wathen gives the history of measures adopted for the relief of lacrymal obstruction, noting that Heister advocated making a hole in the lacrymal bone with a trocar and inserting a tube into the nose through the hole so formed. There is a good description of the anatomy of the parts and one plate of illustrations to elucidate the instruments he used. He recognised the

* See Wathen's will (p. 115) for the relationship between the two men.

epiphora due to eversion of the lower lid and advises a tonic astringent lotion in such cases. Anel, eighty years before the publication of this pamphlet, had first recommended syringing the sac; and Blizard, about twelve years before Wathen's date, had advised filling "the sac with quicksilver, by the fluxility and gravity of which, he concluded the obstruction might be over-come": he had some successful results. Wathen was accustomed to incise the sac from the surface and pass a probe, of medium size, into the nose *via* the nasal duct; he next inserted his special canula. If properly introduced, "the cone and its shoulder are lodged within the nose, and under the *os spongiosum inferius*; the cervix lies within the bony circle; the cup occupies the inferior portion of the lacrymal sac". The canula was passed on a style which was afterwards withdrawn.

Percivall Pott, in 1758, published a tract in eighty-four pages, octavo, on lacrymal fistula. He gives a good description of the anatomy of the parts and with regard to the treatment of lacrymal obstruction lays down three varieties of the disease: (1) Simple dilatation of the sacculus and obstruction of the nasal duct, without any inflammation, and the discharge (upon pressure) of a mucus either quite clear or a little cloudy. (2) Inflammation, abscess, or ulceration of the same parts with the discharge of a purulent mucus, or of matter. (3) Obliteration of the natural duct, attended some-times with caries of the bone. In discussing the first of these, he makes mention of Anel's syringe and probe, and speaks of an instrument invented by Fabricius ab Aquapendente, which was contrived to make pressure over the sac. In the second of his postulates he says there is no remedy without opening the sac-culus; this should be done, if possible, before the sac bursts. If simple incision and fomentations do not bring about a cure, it becomes necessary to dilate the nasal duct. For the third of his postulates he recommends the formation of an artificial passage to the interior of the nose through the os unguis. The ancients, including, apparently, Mr Cheselden, used the actual cautery for making this perforation, but Pott advises a curved trocar.

Mr Phipps tells us that "Mr Wathen attended with the late Mr Gattiker (*sic*) most of the late Baron de Wenzel's operations for a considerable time after his introduction into this country". The Baron's practice was to keep patients flat on their backs for a fortnight or three weeks, on a fluid diet. The eyes were dressed with rags continually wetted with weak brandy and water, and were not inspected till the expiration of that period. Phipps appears to have been in partnership with Wathen. His practice was to uncover the eyes the day after the operation and substitute a shade for the bandage. He relates a few cases in support of this method of treatment.

Wathen's other tract is of 166 pages, octavo. It is entitled:

A | Dissertation | on the | Theory and Cure | of the | Cataract: | in which the practice of | Extraction | is supported; | and that Operation, in its present | improved state, is particularly described: | by Jonathan Wathen, Surgeon. | *Radicitus tollit.* | London: | Printed for T. Caddell, in the Strand; and | C. Dilly, in the Poultry. | MDCCLXXXV. |

It was not until the early years of the eighteenth century that cataract was shown, by dissection, to be "not a pellicle in the aqueous humour in front of the lens, but the opake lens itself, by Maitre Jan (1707), Brisseau (1709) and Heister (1711)". Wathen describes the symptoms and signs and insists on the impossibility of curing cataract by medical means. He lays down excellent rules for the diagnosis of the condition, and as to whether the case is ready for operation. He deprecates the practice of operating in cases of uni-ocular cataract. He describes the old operation of couching and then that of extraction, which Daviel began to practise in 1745. The latter, in 1752, was able to report 206 cases, in 182 of which sight was restored. Sharp's method of operating is next alluded to, the results of which Wathen considers satisfactory. Wathen appears to have followed Sharp's methods in the incision, but he incised the capsule with the "kistitome" of M. de la Faye. The extraction was a simple one, for no iridectomy was performed. He fixed the eye with his finger, helped by an assistant, contrary to the practice of Sharp, who relied upon the steadfastness of the patient.

Wathen died at East Acton, on January 17th, 1808, aged 79.

Mr Wathen Phipps is almost certainly the Watkin Phipps, mentioned in the Farington Diary, as having treated the artist.

The will of Jonathan Wathen is a formidable document of many folio pages. Its chief interest for my purpose is that it clears up some of the uncertainty about Mr Phipps. The following abstract must suffice:

(P.C.C., Ely, 156.)

JONATHAN WATKEN of Upper Berkley St., Portman Sq., May 24th, 1805.

Dwelling house in Berkley Sq. held on lease to wife Elizabeth, with £1,000, all my plate, linen, china, glass, books, pictures and furniture therein; carriages, horses and harness, watches, diamonds, rings and trinkets and wearing apparel.

To brother-in-law Thomas Smith, nephew Samuel Watken and the Rev. Henry Wise, Rector of Charlwood, Surrey £100 each.

To Jonathan Watken Phipps, grandson of my former wife, £300 annuity and three shares in the Sierra Leone Compy. To Catherine Truster, my servant, £20. To Miss Margaret Blackwell my tontine in a chapel at Bath and all my estate therein. To said Thos. Smith, Sam. Watken and Henry Wise £89. 2. 0 long annuities, on trust to pay Miss Hesther Coupe £50 a year for life and Miss Susan and Miss Sarah Watken of King's Stanley, Worcester £10 a year and to Mr Gow now living in Kingsland Road £12. 12. 0 a year and to Mrs Martha Marlborough of near Lisson Green £10, and Mrs Ryland, a poor woman living in Islington, £6. 10. 0. All other freehold lands etc. to the said trustees to sell the same and buy stock and pay dividends to his wife as long as she is a widow; then to his children or child. In the event of these failing he gives long directions as to how his estate is to be partitioned. One share of the ten parts to be paid to Jonathan Watken Phipps and Elizabeth, his wife and their children. Brother-in-law Thos. Smith and nephews Sam. and Nathaniel not to be pressed to repay monies due. Witnesses, Joseph Borrett, Chas. Carr, Rd. Webb Jupp.

A codicil dated 1 March, 1806 deals with the share of nephew Samuel and his children, the "eldest son excepted, as he has a freehold estate under the will of his grandfather, Joseph Watken late of New House, Gloucester, but having seen the will I find this is not so; he is therefore to have his share".

Proved in London, 1 Feb. 1808, by Thomas Smith and Samuel Watken.

It will be noted that he calls himself "Watken" throughout and not Wathen.

GEORGE CHANDLER

The date of Chandler's birth has not been ascertained, but he became a Member of the Corporation of Surgeons in 1769; he was surgeon to St Thomas's Hospital and had much to do with the College of Surgeons. Thus he was elected an Assistant in 1791 and an Examiner and Member of the Court of Assistants from 1800 to 1822. He was Master of the College in 1801, 1808 and 1817, being elected in October of the last named year to fill the vacancy caused by Sir James Earle's death. He practised in Stamford Street and published a *Treatise on the Diseases of the Eye, with its Anatomy, and the Theory of Vision* in octavo, in 1780. In Sprengel's *History of Medicine*, vol. xviii (1820), the book is severely criticised; it is said to be a compilation of little value, a copy in parts from St Yves, Heister and others, and not even a correct copy. Mr South says of Chandler: "He was short in person, bald and grey-bearded, somewhat careless about dress, which was nevertheless scrupulously clean, and in summer time he delighted to appear in nankeen trousers, and was evidently the remnant of an old beau. In manner he was kind and affable to all, even to the poorest person". As an examiner he was popular among the students because of his leniency. "As to his surgical attainments he was a fair surgeon, and personally took as much care of his hospital patients as he would of the most wealthy in private. I often saw him operate, and doubt not that at an earlier period he had been a very good operator, though he was not much of an anatomist. He was very rapid—indeed the quickness with which he operated was marvellous, and appeared almost like conjuring."

Besides the book alluded to above Chandler published *A Treatise of the Cataract, its nature, species, causes and symptoms. With copper plates. By George Chandler, Surgeon. London,* printed for Cadell, 1775. I have not seen a copy of this little book and only know of it from Hirschberg, who says it is an octavo of 116 pages.

I have a copy of his other book and have already abstracted the description of Warner's operation for cataract from it. It is composed of two parts. The first deals with anatomy, the theory of vision, imperfect sights, such as hemeralopia, myopia, presbytia (hypermetropia) and presbyopia; oblique sightedness and squint. The second part is a treatise on diseases of the eye; it deals with ptosis, lagophthalmos, ectropium, trichiasis, ancyloblepharum, tubercles or excrescences on the lids (of which he describes a goodly number), ulceration of the lids, lippitudo, epiphora, cancer of the lids, pterygium, or pannus (which he calls nail or web of the eye), lacrymal fistula, ophthalmy in general, phlyctenulae, abscess of the cornea and corneal ulcers, nebulae, staphyloma, hypopion blocked pupils, photophobia (which he ascribes to inflammation of the choroid), cataract, gutta serena, dropsy of the eye (he makes no mention of the increase of tension in such cases), abscess of the eye and cancers of the globe. I am afraid one can only agree with the adverse criticism expressed above and yet Chandler's book is an early attempt to gather up the knowledge of his day into a more or less complete textbook of eye diseases on modern lines. He died in 1822 or 1823, according to the *Centenary Address of Welcome of the Royal College of Surgeons,* from which the above facts about him are abstracted.

So far as I am aware the will of George Chandler has never been published. The following is the abstract:

(P.C.C., Herschel, 361.)

GEORGE CHANDLER, of Stamford St. in Christchurch, Co. Surrey, esq.

By an indenture made between myself and wife Elizabeth of the first part, Elizabeth Easter of Church Lane in St Luke, Chelsea of the other, dated 25 Aug. last I transferred £9,500 3 % annuities standing in our names upon trust to pay my wife £200 yearly and on the death of either to transfer the principal to the other. This deed is ratified. Debts to be paid.

Henry John Chandler of Upham near Bishops Waltham, Co. Hants., esq., Richard Stevens of the Charterhouse, gent., and nephew Barthw. Jeffery of Peckham, esq. to be exors. and trustees. I leave them £300 each: in trust to pay interest to housekeeper Rebecca Roberts for long and faithful service and after her death it shall form part of the residue. To Mrs Ann Stevens my niece, wife of Richard Stevens, all my globes and telescopes and Flamstead's Atlas. To Bartholomew Jeffery Bruster's Encyclopaedia and my Pantalogia. To niece Susanna Jeffery of Peckham my Encyclopaedia Britannica and all the french books. Burder's Bible and Mant's Bible and all botanical and horticultural books and books on divinity to my nephew the Rev. John Chandler of Traton, York, son of my brother Henry John Chandler. The surgical and anatomical books and instruments to Charles Egerton, esq. son of my nephew the Rev. Charles Egerton of Thorneycomb, Devon. To my servant Sarah Southwood £100. All my household goods and personal effects to my wife Elizabeth. Dated 24 September, 1818. Witnesses, Rich. Pittman of Symonds Inn; W. E. Knobel, his clerk.

Codicil. Revoking terms of legacy to Rebecca Roberts and leaving part to Sarah her daughter and leaseholds at Pig Hill, Sydenham Common to Rebecca absolutely. Dated 1 October, 1818. Witnesses as above. Proved by Richard John Samuel Stevens and Bartholomew Jeffery. 31 July, 1822.

The year of Chandler's death is almost certain to have been 1822.

WILLIAM ROWLEY

We learn from Munk's *Roll* that Rowley was of Irish extraction, and was born in London, in 1743. He was bred a surgeon, and in that capacity served at Belleisle and Havana. He is not included in Johnson's *Roll of Army Medical Service*, so I suppose he was not commissioned. He began life after his military service as a surgeon in London; and in 1774 became M.D. St Andrews. Ten years later he was admitted a Licentiate of the College of Physicians. He also entered at the University of Oxford and became B.A. in 1784; M.A. in 1787; and M.B. in 1788. He was physician to the Marylebone Infirmary and consulting physician to the Queen's Lying-in Hospital. He died in Savile Row, March 17th, 1806, and was buried in St James's Chapel, Hampstead Road.

Rowley was a determined opponent of vaccination and a prolific author; Munk says that his writings "are popular in style, addressed to the public rather than to the profession; and calculated to promote his own interests rather than the science and art he practised. His books have long fallen into complete and deserved oblivion". Munk lists no fewer than twenty-one of his writings. The only one that need concern us is his *Essay on Ophthalmia, or Inflammation of the Eyes and the Diseases of the Transparent Cornea*, published, in octavo, in London, in 1771. This seems to have run through several editions. I have a copy with the following extended title:

A | Treatise | on | One Hundred Diseases | of the | Eyes and Eyelids, etc. | in which are communicated | Several New Discoveries | relative to the | Cure of Defects in Vision; | with many Prescriptions. | by | William Rowley, M.D. | Member of the University of Oxford, the Royal | College of Physicians in London, etc. | To which are added | Directions in the Choice of Spectacles. | London: | Printed for J. Wingrave, (late Nourse's) Strand; | E. Newberry, Corner of Ludgate Hill; and | T. Hookham, New Bond Street. | MDCCXC. |

The preface states that this book is the continuation of those "improvements that commenced above twenty years ago, and were published under the titles, first, of an essay, and afterwards as a Treatise, on the principal Diseases of the Eyes". He speaks of the deceptive pretensions of itinerant oculists, and the neglect of regular practitioners. His introduction occupies sixty-six pages and contains some plates of illustration, the anatomy and physiology and the various methods of treatment in use, some of which he is pleased to commend; in other cases he disagrees and gives his reasons. He is particularly severe upon scarifying and speaks of Woolhouse's scarifier, which was made of beards of wheat.

He gives an account of the operation of excision of the eye which may be included here. The instruments used are "a dissecting knife of a convex or straight form; a pair of scissars with blunt points, a little curved, similar to Daviel's; crooked needles with waxed threads. The dressings include, pledgets of lint of various dimensions; compresses; bandage of rollers; agaric and *spiritus terebinthinae vel vini*". "The patient should sit on a high chair towards the light, and the head should be held back by an assistant. The surgeon stands before the patient. He makes an incision with a straight knife on the junction of the external palpebra with the globe of the eye. The assistant then raises the superior eyelid. The *membrana conjunctiva* is then divided, which connects the superior eyelid with the globe of the eye, near the upper margin of the orbit. The inferior eyelid being well depressed, the conjunctive membrane is to be cut through near the inferior orbital margin, and the bulb of the eye is to be separated from the inferior eyelid. Then by the means of a crooked needle armed with a waxed thread, and passed through the anterior part of the eye, the globe of the eye may be drawn forth from its socket. After the globe of the diseased eye is drawn externally, the fat and muscles are to be separated carefully from the orbit with a crooked knife or scissars. After the separation of the bulb, the optic nerve is to be divided with a crooked knife or scissars, and the whole diseased bulb removed." Since the operation is described for malignant disease, "the surgeon then should carefully examine if there be more indurated or diseased parts remaining, that they may be likewise separated and removed. The cavity of the orbit is then to be filled with lint, over which are to be applied proper compress and bandage: the dressings to remain three days. Then the wound is to be digested and incarned with yellow basilicon, *linimentum Arcaei*, or any other digestive ointment, until the orbit be sufficiently filled to admit the application of an artificial eye". The latter may be of glass or, better, of gold, painted to resemble the other eye.

One more extract from the final section on the application of spectacles may be permitted. "A person formerly applied to me who had a convexity of the cornea, that formed a conic point like the top of a sugar loaf, which no glasses could remedy. This remarkable case happened from the force of crying loud in a hard labor." This was evidently a case of conical cornea.

Rowley's will was proved in London, March 31st, 1806, before Samuel Pearce, parson, Doctor of Laws, Surrogate, by Ann Mary Dunn, spinster, executrix.

This is the will of me William Rowley of Savile Row, St James's, Westminster, Doctor in Physic which I make in manner following (that is to say) I devise all my freehold messuage in old Burlington Street, No. 17 in the occupation of Mrs Legge unto and to the use of George Webb who is now educating at my expense and usually lives with me when in London for and during his natural life and I devise all that my other Freehold Messuage in old Burlington Street No. 16 in the occupation of Edward Sharman unto and to the use of Maria Webb sister of the said George Webb for and during her natural life and as to all the rest and residue of my real and personal estate and also the said two Freehold Messuages after the respective deaths of the said George Webb and Maria Webb I give devise and bequeath the same unto and to the use of Mrs Ann Mary Dunn who now doth live with me and hath for many years past her heirs executors overseers and assigns for ever. And I appoint the said Ann Mary Dunn the sole executrix of this my will. And I do hereby revoke all former wills. Witness my hand and seal this 14th day of March 1806. Wm. Rowley. Witnesses, Robt. Hooper, Elizabeth Hyde, Wm. Seymour.

With the account of Rowley I bring to an end my studies in the history of orthodox ophthalmology prior to the year 1800, leaving only a chapter on the ophthalmic quacks. But in conclusion it is necessary to mention that the year 1794 saw the publication, by John Dalton, of the history of his colour blindness. This is a scarce book. Although Turberville of Salisbury had noted the case of a young woman who saw no colours save black and white, so far as I know no further additions to the subject of colour blindness were made in England until Dalton described his own case.

CHAPTER VIII

The Eighteenth Century (*contd.*)

THE OPHTHALMIC QUACKS

SAMUEL JOHNSON defines a quack as "a boastful pretender to arts which he does not understand"; and in regard to the medical profession, "as one who proclaims his own medical abilities in publick places". The ancients called their quacks *Agyrtae* from the Greek word for a swindler.

Irregular practitioners in the healing arts were recognised by the Act 34–35 Henry VIII, whereby it was lawful for any person being the King's subject, being no common surgeon, but having knowledge and experience of the nature of herbs, roots and waters, etc., to practise and minister medicines to any outward sore and for the stone, strangury, and ague, notwithstanding any Statute to the contrary. This Act became known as the Quack's Charter; it is still unrepealed.

Human nature, being what it is, has enabled the quack to flourish in all ages, and the eye has always been a happy hunting ground for such practitioners. No one will question the statement that the eighteenth century was the heyday of ophthalmic quackery. Sir William Read, who was knighted by Queen Anne, set the fashion in high places, and was followed by Roger Grant and the whole tribe of the Chevalier Taylor; Grant, the Chevalier and at least one of his descendants were royal oculists; and Coats was right when he said that eighteenth-century royalty was singularly unfortunate in its ophthalmology.

Sir William Read flourished from about 1675 till his death in 1715; he was succeeded by Roger Grant; each of these men was illiterate. Read was the son of a Suffolk cobbler and apparently could not even sign his name, while Roger Grant rested his pretensions to practise ophthalmology on the fact that he had lost an eye in the Emperor's service in the continental wars; thus reversing the case of the gladiator alluded to by Martial (*Epigrams* 8. 74):

> *Oplomachus nunc es, fueras ophthalmicus ante.*
> *fecisti medicus quod facis oplomachus.*

The Chevalier Taylor not only surpassed most of the charlatans of his own or any other day, but was a very remarkable man besides. His son and grandson were not of the same calibre. The family has been most ably dealt with by the late George Coats in the last volume of the *Royal London Ophthalmic Hospital Reports*; and his papers are reprinted here by the wish of the editorial committee of the *British Journal of Ophthalmology*. An article by S. Wood, of the library staff of the Royal College of Surgeons, amplifies Coats's article on the Chevalier and should be consulted by those who wish to obtain a fuller knowledge of the man. *Vide British Journal of Ophthalmology*, vol. XIV.[*]

In 1921 I contributed an account of Sir William Read to the *Transactions of the Ophthalmological Society of the United Kingdom*; and a recent paper by Arnold Sorsby, in the *British Journal of Ophthalmology*, vol. XVI, June 1932, has cleared up some difficulties with regard to the book which passes under Read's name.

Contemporary records of the man are meagre in the extreme; they consist of his advertisement, *Post Nubila Phoebus, Nihil absque Deo*, a copy of which is preserved at the British Museum, and various references in the *Spectator* (no. 547) and the *Tatler*. His advertisement was issued from York Buildings, Strand, in 1694; and his *Tatler* advertisement, which appeared soon afterwards, drew public attention to the fact that he had been couching for cataracts for thirty-five years, cutting off wens, curing wry-necks and hare-lips without blemish.

In 1705 Read was appointed Oculist in ordinary to Queen Anne. The warrant of appointment was not found in the "State

---

[*] The author of this paper gives a transcript of a manuscript in the Stone Collection at the Royal College of Surgeons, which seems to have been unknown to Coats. The MS. is in French and deals with the case of the Princess Nariskin.

Papers Domestic" of the period; but the notice appeared in the *London Gazette* of July 30th, 1705, that Read had been knighted on July 27th for his great services done in curing great numbers of soldiers and seamen gratis. Probably some of his combatant patients may have served at Blenheim and at the capture of Gibraltar.

In 1705 appeared a poem in honour of Sir William Read, entitled "The Oculist". This is a small quarto pamphlet of twelve pages, copies of which are at the British Museum and the library of the Royal Society of Medicine; it is a horribly eulogistic affair.

Read's book is a scarce item. Sorsby was able to find only three copies in the medical libraries in London. The copy which I used in writing my paper was entitled:

A | Short but Exact | Account | of all the | Diseases | Incident to the | Eyes | with the | Causes, | Symptoms and Cures. | also | Practical Observations upon some | Extraordinary Diseases of the | Eyes. | by Sir William Read, Her Majesty's Oculist, | and Operator in the Eyes in Ordinary. | The Second Edition, Corrected. | London: Printed, and Sold by | J. Baker, at the Black-Boy in Pater-Noster- | Row. Price, Bound in calf, 2s. 6d. |

Sorsby has proved that the greater part of this book is simply a copy of part of the earlier work in Banister's book, which Read appropriated without acknowledgements. His own part of the book consists of forty pages describing his own wonderful results at the end of it. The copy in the library of the Royal College of Surgeons has a subsidiary title-page which has no printer's name, but gives the date 1706. Sorsby is of the opinion that a second edition was never printed, "the remains of the first and only edition being done up to bring out a second edition corrected".

The book contains an abbreviated edition of Banister's breviary, a practically complete reprint of Guillemeau's book in English, and forty pages of Read's puffs. This latter part was the work of an amanuensis, for Read was unable to read or write.

On April 11th, 1711, Swift wrote to Stella: "Henley would fain engage us to go with Steele, Rowe and others to an invitation of Sir William Read; surely you have heard of him, he has been a mountebank and is the Queen's oculist. He makes admirable punch and treats you in golden vessels".

Read died at Rochester in May 1715 and was buried in the cemetery of St Nicholas in that city. His widow continued his business in Durham Yard, Strand.

Le Neve's *Pedigrees of the Knights* (Harleian Society, VIII, 490) gives the notice from the gazette and ends: "Mem. He was a mountebank formerly servant of Penteus, he was a barbour at Ashdon in Essex, had no right to arms, but bore by usurpation the common coat of Read—Azure a griffon, segreant".

The pedigree is as follows:

Read of Halesworth in Suff. Showmaker = dau'r of —.
Liveing at Halesworth, 1705 and mentioned by her son.

Sir William Read, Liveing in Durham Yard, the oculist.
Dyed at Rochester. = 2nd wife, dau'r of —.

His estate, for he died intestate, was administered by his widow, Augustina, Lady Read.

It will be seen that the greater part of Read's book is about a century out of date. As Sorsby says, the anatomy is that of Galen's time. Some of his puffs may be abstracted in this place.

Read's first puff is entitled "An extraordinary cure of the Gutta Serena, joyned with glaucoma, occuring in one Jeremiah Puttiford, of Watford, deprived of his sight eighteen months, by a violent contusion to the head and right eye". The faculty put his blindness down to a total obstruction of the optic nerves.

Read treated him with cephalics and cordial stomachics. This treatment having produced some slight improvement in the man's condition, and Read having made up his mind that the case was one of glaucoma, he proceeded to treat this with mallows, violets, eyebright, celandine and fennel, together with depletion; he then performed a couching operation and the man received his full sight.

Several cases of cancerous excrescency in the great corner of the eye (the region of the inner canthus) are detailed, one, the case of John Mackleton, of H.M. Horse Grenadiers, who had been wounded thirteen years previously at the siege of Limerick by a musket ball in this region. Read removed the cancer by means of a manual operation, stopped the haemorrhage with his styptic water, prevented the recurrence of the growth by the application of some drying medicines, and in eight days' time restored the patient to his perfect sight.

Another case living at Hayes, near Uxbridge, suffering from a similar condition, was by God's blessing and Read's styptic water, cured after an operation, which cut out the cancer, root and branch. A similar result was obtained in the case of my Lord Mainard's butler, Mr Seedmore.

Mrs Noles, of Hedcox, in Suffolk, suffered from a wen of 10 lbs. weight on her arm; she was cured by means of an operation and the styptic water.

After describing a few cases of cancer of the breast which were cured by operation and the styptic water, Read goes on, "After this digression relating to various cancers, we will now return to the diseases of the eye". He relates the marvellous results of couching in the aged, but enough extracts from this part of the book have been given.

POST NUBILA PHOEBUS. NIHIL ABSQUE DEO.

A sheet about 15 in. by 9 in., printed in two columns on one side only. About one-third of the sheet is occupied by, in the centre, a picture of a patient, and sitting beside him on a seat the quack, in a very full wig, putting into the eye an instrument like a pencil, probably meant for a needle.

An attendant standing on the other side holds the patient's head. On the left side of the picture are: (1) a coat of arms, *viz.* a griffin rampant, impaling a cross ermine, with crest of a demi-

PLATE VII

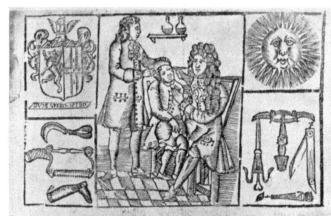

SIR WILLIAM READ'S ADVERTISEMENT

Reproduced from a copy of the original in the British Museum

griffin, and motto, "Dum Spiro Spiro", and (2) below it, small pictures of a curved knife, a saw, and a long boot.

On the right side of the picture are: (1) a sun with human face and rays, and (2) below it, some curious surgical instruments. The above coat of arms bears some resemblance to that of Read, of Llandinan, Co. Montgomery.

The wording of the advertisement is as follows:

These are to give notice, that William Read, Oculist and Chirurgical Operator, being invited by some persons of considerable Quality (who hath been well satisfied of several eminent cures he hath lately performed in the University of Oxford, and this last summer at Windsor) hath encouraged them to send for him, to perform some considerable cures here in Town, as couching of cataracts and curing of cancers, which he frequently performs without cutting, and likewise all Scrophulous Humours, or King's Evil, etc., as many Hundreds in England, Scotland and Ireland can sufficiently demonstrate. He hath been thrice in the University and City of Oxford, where he hath restored Thirty Blind people to their sight by couching, who continue to see very well, which is an operation many pretend to but few perform. He hath a Testimonial from the Vice-Chancellor, for several considerable cures he hath performed in the aforesaid University of Oxford, as upon your further perusal of this Bill you will find, which is a confirmation that he is none of those many Circumforaneus Pretenders that infest this Kingdom: He gives his advice freely, and cures all those that are really poor, of Blindness, Cancers, Wens, Hare-lips, or Wry-necks, gratis, and all others according to his ability, if they come or send to his lodgings while he stays in this Town, which will be for some part of this winter. He hath excellent and approved Remedies to preserve and strengthen the Sight in Young and Old, and to restore hearing, if curable. He likewise infallibly cures all Pains in the Head, that very often occasion the Gutta Serena or Black Cataract, which are never cured, but means may be used in time that may prevent these Obstructions in the Optick Nerves that occasion them. You may have faithful advice of him whether your distempers are curable or not. Out of many cures he hath lately Performed he will only mention these Few, couch'd by him at Oxford in 1689. And at his second coming in 1693, viz. Mrs Souch, Mrs Hall, Mrs Bishop, Mrs Sherlock, Mrs Sawyer, Mrs Simms, Mrs Kerby, Mrs Day, Mrs Faulkner, Mrs Bostel,

Thomas Alcock, Thomas Cliff, Margaret Gole, and many poor People gratis: all restored to their sight.

Captain Cook of Cirencester restor'd by him to his perfect sight although almost Fourscore years of age; and many more in the same countrey.

Hannah Ayres and Alice Ayres, both of the Parish of Denton near Alisbury in Buckinghamshire, were restored to their sight by him, although Blind from their cradles. Madame Strickland of the same Town, who was Blind, was likewise restored to her sight by couching; performed in the year 1693–4.

Windsor, April, 1694. He couch'd Mr Reeves, a gentleman of considerable quality, and restored him to his perfect sight, although Fourscore Years of age: and several others at the same time and Place.

He also Perform'd a very considerable cure, by cutting out a Cancer, which weigh'd ten pounds, from the Breast of Mrs Cary, wife to Mr Ralph Cary, who was servant to King Charles the Second and now liveth at the Blew-Posts in Windsor: This was Perform'd and the Breast preserv'd in its proper shape, by the application of his much approved Styptick-Water, which no man in Christendome truly prepares but himself, although counterfeited by several Ignorant Pretenders that know nothing of the Preparation of it.

Windsor, May 10, 1694. In the Presence of several Persons of Quality, he cut and cured Mrs Mary Glover, the Minister's daughter of Burnham, of a Wry-Neck, contracted down to her Shoulder. And a monstrous Double Hare-Lip for Thomas Goddard of the same Parish.

May 16th, 1694. He couch'd the daughter of Mr John Hanson, Register of Eaton Colledge near Windsor, who was born Blind, and brought her to see very well in a few minutes.

July 14th, 1694. He cut off a mortified Legg from Mrs Ann Crook at Windsor, which was perform'd in half a minute without the loss of an Ounce of Blood after the Styptick-Water was applied; in the Presence of his Grace the Duke of Northumberland.

A Cataract couched by him for the daughter of Mr Johnson at Grundon in Northamptonshire, who was Born Blind, and Restored to her perfect sight; and 20 more in the same countrey in 1687.

John Davenore near Rippon in Yorkshire, although Born Blind, was couched by him, and restored to his perfect sight: and near 100 more in the North of England in the Year 1687 and 1688.

Mrs Joice Wildah of Bath was cured by him in 1693 of a Tympany and Dropsey, when her Belly was as big as a Woman's with Two Children, and he made a perfect cure of it in six weeks without tapping.

A Throat Rupture of a great bigness was cured by him for a Person of considerable Quality in this City.

John Moor of Ogborne near Marlborough in Wiltshire had a large Wen cut off by him from his Belly, which weighed 24 Pound, and he perfectly cured him.

Mrs Whiting near Market-Laventon he cur'd in the year 1693 of a dangerous cancerated Breast without cutting. She was Recommended to him by the Right Honourable the Earl of Abingdon, when left off by all others.

He cut off a very large Cancerated Breast from the Body of Elizabeth Hopkins of Oxford in 1689, and perfectly cured her: for that and many other considerable cures he hath a Testimonial from the Vice-Chancellor.

A French Gentleman belonging to Collonel Cornwal had his skull Trepann'd which was dangerously Fractur'd by a Fall from a Horse, and was cur'd by him at Bath in May, 1693.

He cur'd the wife of John Web of Wooten-Basset in Wiltshire of a Dead Palsie and Convulsion in the Nerves after being eleven years Bed-ridden, and restor'd her to the perfect use of her limbs.

A Wry-Neck contracted down to the Shoulder, cut and cured by him in three days for the daughter of Mrs Cooper at Frome in Somersetshire.

A large deformity of a double Hair-Lip cut and cur'd by him in five days for the son of Mr John Tower, a Merchant of Watchet in Somersetshire.

A Gentlewoman near Guilford in Surrey was cur'd by him of a very dangerous Leprosie. And a child of Mr John Bartlet the Oxford-Carrier, of the same distemper, and both remain in perfect health.

A Polipus in both nostrils, which is an excrescence of Flesh that proceeds from the Brain, was extracted from Mrs Smith at Barnstable in Devonshire in the year 1692, and cured by him in three days.

He is to be spoken with at Mr Agutters a Musical Instrument-Maker at the Sign of the Crown, over-against York Buildings in the Strand, from 8 in the morning till 6 in the evening, where you will see a Bill of Operations hang at the door.

WILLIAM CROSSE

Very little would appear to be known about Crosse. His little book is in 16mo, of 132 pages. The title is a long one, of which the most relevant portion is *A Brief Treatise of the Eyes*. The remainder is concerned with anatomy and diseases, to which are added particular directions for preserving the sight, together with a glossary explaining the terms used. By William Crosse. Practitioner of Physick and Oculist. Printed and Sold by .Morphew, near Stationers' Hall. 1708. Price, bound 1s.

This title-page has a most suspicious appearance of being addressed to the general public, for no one writing for the benefit of his professional brethren would have dreamt of inserting a glossary, which occupies twenty pages, to explain the meaning of the terms he uses. His preface, dated February 4th, 1708, "From my house against Cecil St. in the Strand" does nothing to allay our suspicions; in fact it rather increases them. He inveighs against pretenders, some of whose cases, dismissed by them as incurable, have "since been restored to sight by me". He has drawn upon the works of others for his facts, mentioning Briggs, Keyl, Gibson, Drake and Coward; he also mentions Willis, Sir Theodore Mayerne, Riverius and Coward in speaking of that part of the book which deals with the diseases. He glories in the fact that in this treatise he has omitted to mention the receipts for the medicines which he uses in the cure of cases, lest if they were improperly made use of, "the disappointment of cure would have wholly center'd in me". And so all and sundry with eye complaints are adjured to call on him, where they will meet with candid and fair treatment.

Crosse uses the term iris for the limbus in discussing the insertions of the recti muscles, just as Turberville did with regard to the situation of a particle of steel stuck in the cornea. He repeats the remarks of Briggs in dealing with the obliques and even the quotation from the *Aeneid*, of which he offers a translation of his own. The rest of the book consists of short accounts of the following ophthalmic conditions: gutta serena; suffusion or incipient cataract; ophthalmia, under which heading we are informed of the great value of his specific powders in rectifying the disorders of the blood and juices, and the virtue of his specific eye wash; albugo and specks; hypopion; phlyctenulae; corneal ulcers; aegilops, or fistula lacrymalis; epiphora and pterygion.

It would seem that the book is scarce. Hirschberg notices it and states that no copy exists in German libraries, or in the Bowman Library of the Ophthalmological Society. I am indebted to the librarian of the Royal Society of Medicine for the loan of their copy. It is sad stuff.

As to the author it is just possible, though I do not think it very likely, that he may have been the William Crosse mentioned by Foster in *Alumni Oxonienses* (first series, vol. 1) as the son of Benjamin, of Cork, Ireland, cler. He was of St John's College and matriculated April 29th, 1692, aged 16. B.A. 1695/96; B.Med. 1705; D.Med. 1706. Admon. (at Oxford) September 13th, 1709. As this word "Admon." refers to the administration of the estate of an intestate, it would appear that he did not live long to reap the reward of his disinterested advice to the reader. The following letter, Sloane MS. 4058, fol. 202, may possibly be from Crosse to Sir Hans Sloane. It looks as if the writer were in low water:

May it please your Hon'

As gratitude has me under the striktess oblygation of acknowledging the favour I have already received from you So thinking myself oblyged to inform you That after I had pay'd my respects first to you as President. I then waited on several of the Worthy Members who advised me to apply myself to yr Hono' in this manner And that if you was then pleased to espouse my Interest they would contribute to my relief. Might I trespass so far on yr goodness I should want words to express my Thanks for so great a Favour confer'd on me.

Yr Hono^r

Most Humble and

most obedient Servant

WM CROSSE.

One other letter of William Crosse, at the British Museum, is not in the same hand.

CHAPTER IX

The Chevalier Taylor*

BY GEORGE COATS

IN the eighteenth century ophthalmology had not yet vindicated, in England, its position as a separate branch of practice. It was the province of a set of ambulant practitioners who toured the country accompanied by all the apparatus of shameless advertisement (including "monkies", we are told), couching cataracts, and selling infallible salves and eye washes. This taint of quackery appears to have deterred respectable surgeons from meddling much with the subject; their operative experience was probably small, and the procedure of couching, attended frequently with brilliant immediate, but disastrous after results, was likely to be performed with fewer scruples by itinerant oculists, here to-day and gone to-morrow, than by settled practitioners who had to abide the consequences of their handiwork.

Among these travelling quacks the name of the "Chevalier" Taylor stands pre-eminent for unblushing effrontery, blatant self-laudation, and all the methods of the charlatan, but also for mental endowments far above the average of his tribe, and for a real acquaintance with the contemporary state of ophthalmic knowledge. His fame extended to every country in Europe; his boast of having conversed with kings and princes is no idle one; he had an acquaintance, not always felicitous, with some of the best-known men, medical and lay, of his time; counting translations and minor works he was the author of nearly fifty books; and in later life he wrote an autobiography, which, if it gives few and unreliable particulars as to his actions, does much to reveal the character of the man.

* Published in the *Royal London Ophthalmic Hospital Reports*, vol. xx, p. 1, May 1915.

PLATE VIII

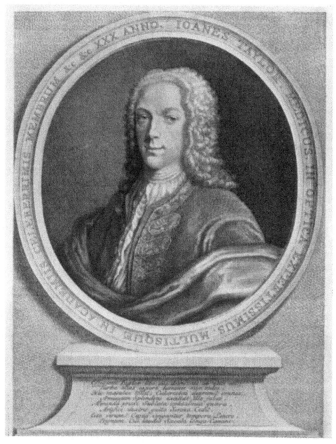

THE CHEVALIER TAYLOR

Reproduced from a print in the British Museum

In justification of the resumption of a subject which has been dealt with from a general or special standpoint by Stricker, Schrön, Norrie, Antonelli, Frank, Hirschberg and v. Duyse, it may be pleaded that no English account of Taylor's life and works has appeared, that a considerable number of English sources have never been fully tapped; and especially that no recent writer seems to have had access to the *Travels and Adventures*(19)* which forms the basis of much of the first section of this paper.

LIFE AND CHARACTERISTICS

It was in Norwich that the Chevalier, to quote his own phrase, "first became acquainted with the glories of the sun", and he more than hints that the town will one day be famous on that account. The date was August 16th, 1703, the hour, as a medal struck in his honour informs us, eleven in the forenoon.† His ancestors, he says, were eminent in divinity and physic, his father in the latter. It was in a mood of unwonted modesty, however, that he wrote this; elsewhere he claims to be noble, not only from his rare acquirements, but also by birth(88), and states that he was born in a land where nobility is no bar to the practice of a scientific calling(96). The truth is that his father was John Taylor, surgeon, of Norwich, who died about 1709.‡ The social

* These figures, throughout this work, refer to the Bibliography and References at p. 193.

† "Between eleven and one", says the spurious Life and History. The alternative date, October 13th, 1708, given by some authors, is certainly wrong. See his family tree published in *Norfolk Archaeology* (87). As Hirschberg (84) has pointed out, it is unlikely that Taylor should have written the *Mechanism of the Eye* in 1727 at the age of nineteen.

‡ "An eminent surgeon at Norwich, and highly respected in his private, as well as his professional, character", says the Chevalier's grandson (97). I do not know on what authority Schrön (94) says that he was the son of the "considerable mathematician, Brook Taylor, Doctor of Laws". There were five generations of John Taylors, of whom four followed a medical career, and three were oculists. The Chevalier's only son succeeded to his practice and died in 1787; his grandson was Oculist to George III and George IV, and died in 1832, aged 76. A brother of the Chevalier, the Rev. Jas. Taylor, A.M., was Rector of Broadway in Dorset, and a Chaplain to George II, and to His Majesty's Own Regiment of Horse. He published a work on the German Empire.

position of the family seems to have been fairly good; a collateral branch acquired by marriage Breccles Hall, a considerable estate in Norfolk(87).

Following always, be it understood, his own account, he was bred to general practice, went regularly through every branch of his profession under the best masters in England,* attended the practice of St Thomas's Hospital regularly and diligently, as Cheselden will bear witness, passed his examinations "with all becoming exactness", and, while scarcely of age, was appointed chief surgeon to one of the most important provincial hospitals in England—Norwich Hospital, it may be presumed(19).

In his earliest work we hear of his having "cut for the stone", but almost from the first his attention was directed towards his future speciality, and during his "infant days", he wrote a *Treatise on the Eye*, which fell under the notice of Dr Desaguliers of Cambridge. That gentleman at once recommended him to become a specialist, pointing out—truly enough, apparently— that there were no oculists who had undergone a complete training in other branches of medicine. Unfortunately for the credibility of this account, however, the Chevalier attributes this advice later in the same work to Petit.† Fired by these praises he determined to put the doctor's recommendation into practice, but before doing so resolved to extend his experience by travel.

Accordingly in 1727 he set out, touring first through England,

---

* The fact that his father was a surgeon gives an increased air of probability to this relation, and, indeed, his books show a good medical knowledge. The statement(91) that he was educated at Cambridge seems to be erroneous. He could scarcely have escaped some tincture of classical learning, of which he had none, if he had attended that University.

† But again the claims of Dr Desaguliers are reinforced—or, if the reader pleases, the whole tale is discredited—by the fact that it is open to grave doubt whether the Chevalier, as late as 1765, had ever met Petit. In that year we find Dr Marteau, of Amiens, writing to Petit that Taylor "me temoigne le plus grand empressement de faire connaissance avec vous, je me fais un plaisir de lui en fournir l'occasion" (80). This seems to dispose of the story, mentioned by Hirschberg (84), that Taylor makes no mention of his journey to Paris in 1734 because he had stolen Petit's method of operating for cataract. In fact, the journey to France *is* mentioned in the *Travels and Adventures*.

Scotland, Ireland and Wales, and returning to London in 1733, where he remained until March 1734.* The following account of his subsequent movements is founded on Taylor's own itinerary, as given in the *Travels and Adventures*(19), but with some very necessary corrections from notices in contemporary periodicals, and where possible from the dates and places of publication of his works. In 1734 he went to France, and is said to have been at Marseilles in that year(90, 94). He travelled through France, Holland, and back to London in 1735. In 1736 he returned to Paris, and from 1737 to 1742 toured through Spain and Portugal, where he is said to have celebrated his greatest triumphs. In 1742 or 1743 he appears at Rouen, and between these years and 1746 he made another circuit of England, Scotland and Ireland. He passed over in 1747 to Holland and Flanders.†

During 1750 he was in Germany. In 1751 he was called to Rostock to restore the sight of the Duke of Mecklenburg-Schwerin, and visited Hamburg and Denmark. In 1752 he was in Sweden. During 1753 and 1754 he travelled day and night,

* Haller seems to bear witness that Taylor attended the lectures of Boerhaave in Leyden during 1725 ((40a), "mecum a. 1725 Boerhaavium audierat"). If so it is very extraordinary that Taylor, boasting, in 1727, of the thoroughness of his medical education, should make no mention of the fact, or should ever state in any of his works that he was out of England before 1734. Perhaps the date may be wrong, but Boerhaave is said to have resigned the chairs of Chemistry and Botany at Leyden in 1729 (*Encycl. Brit.* Art. "Boerhaave"). In later works Taylor claims to have known and consulted with Boerhaave, who at first did not like the treatment which he proposed, but afterwards became converted to his views.

† There is considerable doubt as to this last statement, however, and also as to his movements during the years 1747 to 1749. He himself asserts that he was in Germany, Prussia, Saxony and Vienna during this time. It is certain that he was in Northampton in January 1747 (85), in Edinburgh in April 1749, in Dublin during the summer of 1749 (68), in Amsterdam in September of that year (48), and in Germany in 1750 (4a). Is it likely that he went through Germany as far as Vienna, back to Edinburgh, and once more to Germany in so short a time? For reasons which will be appreciated later, the Chevalier usually allowed a considerable interval to elapse between his visits to any given country. His work throws no light on the point, nothing having been published between 1747 in Edinburgh and 1750 in Germany. On the whole, it is probable that this visit to Germany is fictitious, and that he did not leave Britain between 1747 and 1749.

passing through Sweden, Copenhagen, Breslau, Silesia, Warsaw, Mittau, Courland, Riga, St Petersburg and Moscow. In 1755 he journeyed through Germany and Bohemia. In 1756 he was in Italy. In 1757 he travelled back through Vienna and Ghent, reaching London in 1758 or 1759. During 1759 and 1760 he made another tour through Scotland, Ireland and Wales. In 1761 he was in London "at Gravel St., Hatton Garden"; during this and the following year he published his *Travels and Adventures*, and announced his determination to enjoy a well-earned rest. But the wandering spirit was too strong for him. We catch a glimpse of him in 1765 at Amiens and Rheims(80), and in 1767 at Ghent(81); a work of his was published in Hamburg and Leipzig in 1766(9 e), and on June 6th, 1772, he died in Paris say some authorities—in a convent at Prague according to his grandson's account(97). He is said to have become blind before his death.

His epitaph, composed by himself, is given by Guérin(39), and is in what he calls "his well-known peculiar manner". He has been eager only for the fame of others, has diligently sought the society of the learned, and has found his highest joy in earning their friendship. In addition to some Latin verses used elsewhere in his works, the following stanza is appended:

> Dieux! Taylor gît dans cette bière;
> Cet oculiste si fameux;
> Après avoir donné tant de fois la lumière,
> Devait il donc fermer les Yeux!

The considerable discrepancies between his own account of his itinerary and the facts show that, even when he had presumably no reason or intention to falsify, the Chevalier's word is not to be taken without reserve. It is evident that he was a man totally devoid of what one of Scott's characters calls "a pettifogging intimacy with dates, names, and trifling matters of fact —a tiresome and frivolous accuracy of memory".*

* It will be seen that there is no place here for the journey to Transcaucasia and Persia which Stricker (96) places between 1755 and 1762. Taylor *says*, in 1761, that

During these journeys the Chevalier met and saw everyone and everything of the least consideration in the whole of Europe. Boerhaave "continued me his correspondence and friendship to his latest hours", Haller had "taken extraordinary pains to recommend me to the favour of the public", Morgagni was present when "I was created doctor of Chirurgery in the University of Padua"; Winslow, Hunter, Monro and Linnæus were numbered among his acquaintances. He travelled a hundred leagues to see Metastasio "that no great man might escape me", and for the same reason, presumably, was on speaking terms with those notorious criminals, Jonathan Wild, Jack Sheppard and the Rabbit Woman.*

Honours and diplomas were showered upon him. In 1734, after proving his abilities to the faculty, he was made a Fellow of the College of Physicians of Basel, and degrees were subsequently conferred upon him in Liège, Cologne and Rheims. Innumerable learned societies granted him testimonials or received him as a member. Municipalities presented him with sums of money.†
He held the office of "ophthalmiater" to the Pope, the Emperor, and a multitude of Kings, Electors and Sovereign Princes, whose names may be read in the title-page of some of his works(19).

Among the exalted personages under his care were the Duke of Mecklenburg, the Princess of Georgia, the Countess of

he has been among Tartars, Turks, Hungarians, Georgians and Calmucks, and that he published in 1754 a book on the cure of the Princess of Georgia, "Aunt to Prince Heraclius supposed to be the present Sophy of Persia", but the falseness of his statement and his ignorance of geography are shown by his having once asserted that he travelled to Archangel to meet the prince, Archangel being in the extreme north of Russia, and Georgia a Transcaucasian state (86). Moreover, he certainly published a work in Edinburgh in 1759. His Asiatic travels, therefore, may be regarded as fictitious.

* Mary Tofts, of Godalming, who was supposed to have given birth to seventeen rabbits. Many were deceived, including St André, the King's surgeon. The learned, if heterodox, Whiston wrote a pamphlet to prove that the event was the consummation of a prophecy in Esdras. Her imposture was finally exposed by Sir Thos. Clarges.

† At least one statement to this effect has been definitely refuted (100).

Windischgraz, the illustrious Lady Nariskin, and Don A. de Saldana, Viceroy of the Indies.★

In all this extravagant boasting there is, undoubtedly, a kernel of truth. His objectionable methods were not the growth of a day, and there seems no reason to doubt that he did, in fact, receive degrees from several universities—the smaller ecclesiastical, rather than the larger, more scientific, schools, says Stricker(96). His claim to have been appointed oculist to George II in 1736 is perfectly authentic, as is shown by the following extract, for which I am indebted to the Deputy-Keeper of the Public Records.

Dr Taylor to be sworn Oculist in Ord^{ry} to His Ma^{sty}.   These are, etc., Dr John Taylor into the place and quality of Oculist and Operator for the Eyes in Ord^{ry} to His Ma^{sty}. To have, hold, exercise, and enjoy the said place together with a[ll] rights, profits, priviledges, and advantages thereto belong[ing] and etc. Given, etc., this 21st Day of May, 1736, in the 9th year of His Majesty's Reign.

GRAFTON.

To the Gent Ushers, etc.
[Lord Chamberlain's Appointment Books (L.C. $\frac{3}{65}$).]

In the *Scots' Magazine* for 1744 (p. 344) we read: "Dr Taylor, who has visited Glasgow and is returned, has caused register in the books of council and session, his diplomas as Doctor of Medicine by the Universities of Basel and Rheims in 1734, and by those of Liège and Cologn in 1735; also a certificate of his having been duly admitted oculist in ordinary to His Majesty in 1736".†

★ The notorious Baron de Wenzel is said to have been his pupil, and, if so, evidently learned from him more than the mere dry bones of ophthalmic science (97). He was subsequently preferred to the Chevalier's son in an application for appointment as Oculist to George III.

† The certificate is given in full in the *Travels and Adventures*. His grandson had heard that the Chevalier, on this appointment, had declined to receive the same salary as was allotted to the Poet Laureate (97).

Some of the testimonials or "sentiments" of the learned have perhaps no great internal air of credibility, such as the following from the College of Rome.

As to illustrious patients, his claim is well founded at least in the case of the Duke of Mecklenburg. He certainly treated Gibbon, but does not think fit to include so plebeian a person in his list.* He asserts that he operated on Bach and Handel, the former, "at Leypsick, where a celebrated master of music, who had already arrived at his 88th year, received his sight at my hands"; in Handel's case he hoped to have the like success, "but, upon drawing the curtain, we found the bottom defective, from a paralytic disorder". These statements contain a good average of inaccuracies. First, Bach never did attain his 88th year; second, he did not receive his sight, but became blind after operation; third, Handel's operation was performed by William Bromfield in 1750, and though the operation was unsuccessful he did not become completely blind. Taylor's ignorance of the whole matter is shown by his assertion that Handel was educated by Bach, whereas, in fact, they never met.

These public and professional triumphs, however, are colourless compared with some of his private adventures. On one occasion a princess disguised herself as a poor girl and stopped him on the roadside, in order to discover if he were truly charitable, an ordeal from which, needless to say, the Chevalier emerged gloriously. At a masked ball he made love to a lady, who after two hours assured him of a "reciprocal return". At the hour of unmasking she stood revealed as the Hereditary Princess of the Court. On another occasion, a princess, fearing that his conversation might be restrained by her august presence,

"In the name of the Lord, Amen. We, the Archiator, physicians, general counsellors, and doctors of this college, from the various testimonies we have of the learning and ability of the illustrious Chevalier John de Taylor, from his knowledge in general in the several branches of physic and surgery, and above all for his marvellous ability in that which regards the eye; we do, by these letters patent receive him with one united heart as a member of our corps, etc."

A selection of such sentiments is given in the form of footnotes to the second volume of the *Travels and Adventures*, and occupies eighty-six pages.

* "From Hans Sloane and Dr Mead, to Ward and the Chevalier Taylor, every practitioner was called to my aid." *Autobiog. of Edw. Gibbon*, ed. J. Murray, 1896, p. 36.

disguised herself as a serving maid, and pretended to be a patient.
The Chevalier, finding her beautiful, at first made love to her,
but afterwards, suspecting her of being of higher rank than
appeared, he began to "play with words", a fashionable accom-
plishment at which he was a great adept. When the identity of
the lady was disclosed Taylor's elegant apology was graciously
received by the princess, who called him "Dear Englishman!
charmer of my heart", and invited him to sup with her.

In affairs of gallantry he was an acknowledged authority, and
was frequently consulted by "very great personages". He tells
us that he "once ventured abroad a little piece in Italian on 'The
Art of making Love with Success'"; and also that "the lady is
not living on this side of forty, but on fixing my eyes upon her,
I can read her very soul". In fact, the wiser the lady the more
likely is she to succumb, because she will be the better able to
appreciate the Chevalier's wit. On one occasion he received an
offer of marriage from a wealthy lady of 90, but discreetly misunderstood her meaning. We have independent testimony,* and
indeed his portraits confirm the fact, that he was a man of good
personal appearance. His grandson also testifies, though not
from personal recollection, that he was "a tall, handsome man,
and a great favourite with the ladies"(97).

His more prosaic adventures were variegated. He had seen
Jews burned, and knew all the secrets of the Inquisition; he had

---

* Dr W. King (59) says "he has a good person", and speaks of him, perhaps not
without a spice of irony, as "vultu compto, corpore procero, fronte urbana
gloriosus", i.e. famed (or ostentatious) for his handsome features, tall person, and
refined countenance (or town-bred face, i.e. assurance, impudence). Beer (78) also
testifies that he was a handsome man (quoted by Hirschberg (84), p. 299). His
portrait, painted by Chevalier Riche in Rome, and engraved by John Faber, Jun., is
prefixed to the Mechanismus des Auges (4); another very good picture of him will be
found in the Racolta dell' opere scritte (30). Taylor's grandson mentions a picture
painted at Rome by "the Chevalier Rosco" which was sent home by Taylor after
he had quitted England for the last time (97). His family held it to be an excellent
likeness. "It represents him in splendid attire, and in a dignified attitude, holding
the instrument for couching in his hand, with an artificial eye, for the illustration of
a lecture which he seems to be delivering."

witnessed the various species of torture and methods of embalming, had studied the practice of inoculation in all lands, had met gipsies and hermits, and conformed to their manner of life. He was robbed on the frontiers of Spain and Portugal, and also between Naples and Rome, where he lost "pictures of crowned heads, incircled with brilliants, instruments of solid gold, etc., to the value of 30,000 Roman crowns", and barely escaped with his life; but he received from the authorities a certificate of his misfortune, which served as an excellent advertisement.

He had a large practice in nunneries and convents, the details of which, he seems to think, must be of superlative interest to English readers. One of his artifices, of which he makes no secret, was to introduce inquisitive young noblemen into the forbidden precincts, in the guise of his assistants; but he plumes himself on never having permitted the least impropriety. On one occasion he held a conversation with a friar who had been down to Hell. Taylor asked him if he had any witnesses. "Witnesses," said he, in the greatest warmth, "you amaze me; would any but an Englishman have talked to me of witnesses in an affair of this kind?" He is said to have given a ball at Dresden, during which he changed his shirt and peruke twenty times, taught the ladies the English contre-dance, and, at the end, attempted to leave without paying the bill (Hirschberg (84), p. 296).

It is very seldom that the touchstone of other evidence can be applied to those fantasias. There is one incident, however, of which we possess an independent account. In 1750 he arrived in Prussia and sent his credentials to Frederick the Great. The authentic account of what followed, as related by the Margravine of Anspach, an English lady, formerly Lady Craven (53), is an excellent instance of the sardonic humour of that king; the version in the *Travels and Adventures* is a no less instructive illustration of some of the Chevalier's characteristics.

An English oculist, [says the Margravine] being at Berlin during Voltaire's residence there, as he was a member and a professor of all the academies in Europe, wished to be admitted to the King, in order to be appointed oculist to His Majesty. The King at that time, for some reason, held the English at arm's length, and was so little desirous of pleasing the country in general that he would hardly be civil to any particular individual of it, though backed with a title or offices of State.

[Here follow various instances of Frederick's incivility.]

At the time the English nobility were thus humiliated and excluded the Court, the Oculist was publicly admitted; and, to render it more satirical against us, with double honour, superior to what a person of that rank deserved, however his usual vanity might desire or expect it. The Doctor was also strongly suspected of being employed by our Ministry as a private observer of the several actions of Princes; and his profession giving him opportunities, he was perpetually fluctuating between one court and another, and admitted to the presence in all. The Oculist being introduced to the King, His Majesty, with his usual politeness, asked him what favours he could confer on him, being ready to distinguish him and all men of his eminence. The Doctor only desired the honour of being appointed Oculist to His Majesty; and which, to make short of, the King granted; adding, "As I do not love to suspend anyone's happiness long, be at Court to-morrow early, and your patent shall be ready". The Chevalier, flushed with this promise, so unexpected, now appeared at Court as by Royal Command; but, notwithstanding a double parade of laqueys and equipage, on his approach to the King, His Majesty said, "You desire to be my Oculist—there is your patent: you must take the usual oaths on these occasions; that done, come to me again". On his reporting to the King that all necessary forms were gone through, His Majesty said, "You desired to be my Oculist—you are so: my eyes want no assistance; yet are you my Oculist; but if you touch the eyes of one of my subjects, I will hang you up. I love my subjects equally with myself". The Chevalier departed, or rather was ordered to depart, in six hours; he pleaded for more time to pack up his eyes and instruments, but was refused; and a guard being set over him, he was then escorted, like any delinquent, to the borders of Saxony—that being the country most contiguous. . . . Voltaire wrote an epigram* on this, the point of which was that the King had driven from his dominions the only man who could have opened his eyes.

Taylor's version of what must be the same incident is that his banishment was due to the inveterate malice of a courtier over

---

* I have been unable to find it in his published works.

whom he had gained a battle of wits. The King's mind having been poisoned by this gentleman, all remonstrances and representations were vain. The crisis was grave, disgrace and loss faced him, but the Chevalier was equal to the emergency. He visited all the principal persons on his list, performed a pretended operation, and applied a bandage. Then, having impressed upon them the many risks of the after-treatment, he informed them that he was banished, and that if their eyes were to be saved they must accompany him to the next country. Accordingly, the next morning he set out in triumphal procession, followed by a brilliant train of equipages, crossed the border into Saxony, and there undertook the cure of his patients and received their thank-offerings. With this tale before us we shall have little difficulty in appreciating the small kernel of truth and the enormous husk of falsehood in most of the Chevalier's anecdotes.*

Several passages in the *Travels and Adventures* make us acquainted with the Chevalier's views on such subjects as the art of pleasing, prejudice, happiness in marriage, suicide, duelling, jealousy, despotism; all these being illustrated by a wealth of anecdotes in which he either took a prominent part or "knew the man". His prescription for happiness in marriage is to "let both resolve that all each says or does is right". The art of pleasing is to "show the person we are with to advantage". He says, truly it may be presumed, that he has "known marvellous effects from the power of faith". In speaking of religion he drops the mountebank, and for once we seem to listen to his genuine thoughts. "Both opinions [the Protestant and Catholic] are right. . . ; or if you please, which is pretty much the same thing, they are not in the wrong, neither are we." "The ceremony of every religion has its beauties", and they "are all

---

* Yet another version is found in the memoirs of the Chevalier's grandson (97). Frederick "would not permit him to practise in his dominions, alleging that he should take care of the eyes of his subjects himself, that they might see no more than was necessary for the interest and glory of their country. It was, however, understood that the monarch had been told that to admit a foreigner to practise would be throwing an odium on the medical professors of his own territory".

different roads to the same point". He enters a plea for tolera-
tion, yet warns his readers that the young should not be taught
exotic opinions too early, before their own convictions are consolidated. His wandering life has given the same cosmopolitan
note to his patriotism. As to virtues and vices, all nations "differ
only in the manner, but little in the degree". For painting, music
or architecture he prefers Italy, for pleasure other nations, but
"after all I have seen, and after all I have said, I give Britain the
preference, as well for the perfections of the state as the happiness
of the people". But he is not above turning these liberal sentiments to account. In an advertisement of 1752 he tells us that
"he is an Englishman, but without servile preference for his own
nation, a man of learning, but without boasting, and unique of
his kind"(38). On another occasion he repudiates the universally
recognised foibles of his countrymen in the following terms:
"An Englishman without being addicted to drinking, without
an unequal and unsteady temper, without a preconceived
flattering opinion about his nation".

He was a great admirer of the quality, and addressed himself
only to ladies of rank and condition, "for those of the lower
class do not come under my consideration". Elsewhere also he
tells us that the reason of the common people is small, that they
are strangers to argument, and that nothing but the laws can keep
them in bounds.

Of his private manner of life scarcely anything is known. He
married a certain Ann Price(87), but whether she accompanied
his wandering life is uncertain. His grandson(97) informs us that
he was "much addicted to splendour, and to an expensive style
of domestic expenditure". The boy was a favourite with his
grandfather, who "would throw himself on the floor in his rich
attire, suffer me to sit on his breast as if I were on a horse, and
give his laced neckcloth to me to hold as a bridle".

After this exposition of the Chevalier's life and opinions it will
be felt that his apology, "if in any part of this work [the *Travels
and Adventures*] I have forgot the gravity that becomes the

physician and the scholar", is not superfluous. Let us now turn
to his methods.

METHODS

The Chevalier's entry into the towns which he honoured with
his sojourn was scarcely that of a thief in the night. In what he
calls the "crisis of his grandeur" he travelled with "no less than
two coaches and six, above ten servants in livery, besides gentlemen, my companions, in my own pay"(19). It is said, on what
ultimate authority I do not know, that his coach was painted
over with eyes, and bore the motto which occupies the title-page
of nearly all his works *Qui dat videre dat vivere,* or alternatively
Qui visum, vitam dat(88, 96). The spectators who flocked, we are
told, by tens and hundreds to see him, were gratified by a sight
of his valuables, his magnificent array of instruments glittering
with gold, his portfolios of public and private testimonials(47).
In the morning he treated patients, in the afternoon he performed
operations and gave demonstrations; and on Sundays and other
days he delivered special lectures, such as he had given before all
the crowned heads and learned societies of Europe, in praise of
the eye, its beauties, and the art of re-establishing and preserving
vision. To these lectures and also to his demonstrations and operations the nobility, gentlemen, ladies, and more especially the
faculty were invited(85); some meetings were reserved for
ladies(86). He lectured on anatomy with the help of "a most
exquisite piece of workmanship in enamel, intended to represent,
in 325 figures, the several diseases of the globe of the eye"(66, 80,
84). See Appendix I, p. 210.

His arrival was accompanied, and presumably preceded, by
showers of leaflets, placards, and advertisements in the public
press, many of which have been preserved. His epitaph, mentioned above, was put to excellent *ante-mortem* service in this
way(39). Some of these advertisements were merely handbills
announcing the place, date, and subject of his lectures; of these
the following is a good example; another specimen is given in

Appendix I, p. 210, and others are quoted in the *Ann. d'Oc.*(76), and by v. Duyse(81).

Northampton, Saturday, December 19th. To-morrow, being *Sunday*, the 20th (as usual on that day),—the Gentlemen,—the Ladies,—the Clergy, and all of Literature and Distinction, are hereby invited—at Six in the Evening, at the Great ROOM, at the *Red-Lyon* to a *Phisico-Theological Declammation* in Praise of SIGHT, design'd both in Speaking and Action, agreeable to the Rules of ORATORY.—The SYLLABUS—will be given free to all present, and the Whole will be free.—By JOHN TAYLOR, Esq.,—Doctor of Physick,—Oculist to the King of GREAT BRITAIN,—Fellow of several Colleges of Physicians, etc. Being a Specimen of a Course many Years given in the several Universities, and the several Courts abroad—*London, Edinburgh*—and lately at *Dublin. The* Gentry are invited every morning to see his METHOD *of restoring* SIGHT, etc.—At Six on Monday Evening next (the 21st Instant) he will certainly give the LECTURE on the Alterations of the EYE, etc.—When the Eye will be dissected, and all its various Beauties displayed, in the Order of a Work lately published in Octavo, with Plates, at EDINBURGH. Notwithstanding the Many that usually attend on this Occasion, the ROOM will be so regulated that every Person present may see the several Parts of the EYE accurately examin'd.

In an advertisement at Ghent in 1757 he consents, at the instance of diverse persons of condition, to delay his journey to Brussels for a few days in order to render aid to the townspeople. Ten years later he is again delayed in the same town by the large number of persons who flock to him from all parts (v. Duyse(81)).*

Other advertisements, however, evidently directed towards the "gentlemen, ladies, clergy, and all of literature and distinction" above-mentioned, are much more elaborate. In the British Museum there is a work of this type in Italian and German, the *Racolta dell' opere scritte . . . dal Cavaliere Giovanni di Taylor*(30). On the title-page there is an excellent picture of the Chevalier, with some Latin verses beginning, *O! tu, qui terris ades, Esculapius alter*; then follows a catalogue of his works,

---

* I am greatly indebted to Prof. v. Duyse for sending me a copy of his interesting communication, "Les Oculistes ambulants à Gand au 18me Siècle".

two pages of his titles and honours, a list of his patrons, a prospectus of new works to be published, and some testimonials.

Another device was to issue a panegyric in which the name of the author was modestly screened as "one of the most noble and most learned men of our time"(88), or as "Prof. H—, of the University of G—"(38). A good example of this class is entitled *A Parallel between the late Celebrated Mr Pope and Dr Taylor, Oculist to the King of Great Britain, etc., by a Physician*(29). In this work the name of Pope is a mere stalking-horse, and appears only once between the earliest paragraphs and the second last page; both great men were persecuted by ignorance and malice; Pope was precocious in one walk of life, Taylor in another. The rest of the pamphlet is in the usual style. Though yet very young (he was forty-five at the time) he has surpassed all who lived before him, and all contemporaries. The accusation that he travels too fast to give his patients proper attention might apply to an ordinary man, but his method "is not a tedious and dangerous course of Medicine, but by the Hand, where the Event is almost instantly known". As to the rumour that he undertakes hopeless cases, it is true, of course, that he has treated diseases *supposed* to be incurable, but never such as he himself considered to be beyond help; on the contrary, in such cases he has refused "a common Fee for his Opinion, tho' his Right as a Physician". He emphasises the complete safety of his operations —sixty in number—points out that operative dexterity is only to be acquired by practice, and that one might watch a painter for ever without learning to paint; he describes the joy of the operator on drawing the veil "when the Eye, that beauteous, that inestimable, that divine little Globe again its native Power reclaims, again becomes a Lucid Orb". It is as rare for Taylor to have a failure as for others to have a success; his operations are seldom even followed by congestion. Of 243 diseases of the eye formerly not sixty were curable; now not sixty are incurable. He keeps no secrets, and rejoices that his discoveries should be made public. The style of his lectures is elegant, and when ladies are to be particularly addressed he makes it clear that he has seen the best company. The work contains also a poem by "one of the greatest judges living, of that style for which Mr Pope was so justly celebrated", which will be found in Appendix II (p. 211).

What the regular faculty thought of all this belongs to the next section, but the following lay view, contained in a letter dated January 4th, 1747, from one John Palmer to Dr Ducarel, deserves to be transcribed in full(85):

The excessive deep snows, floods, and bad roads, kept me so much at home that, for want of company, I had almost read myself blind by way of amusement; so, to change the scene, about ten days ago I crept over to Northampton, and luckily met there with the famous Dr Taylor, who operated every morning, and read lectures, as he call'd them, every evening to twelvepenny chaps, except on Sundays, when he gave *gratis* a Declamation (as you'll see by this advertisement enclosed, which was delivered to every house in town).* This gratis, I own, took me in for an auditor; and I'll tell you how it was carried on. The Doctor appeared dress'd in black, with a long, light flowing ty'd wig; ascended a scaffold behind a large table raised about two feet from the ground, and covered by an old piece of tapestry, on which was laid a dark-coloured cafoy† chariot-seat, with four black bunches (used upon hearses) tyed to the corners for tossels, four large candles on each side the cushion, and a quart decanter of drinking water, with a half-pint glass, to moisten his mouth. He bowed, snuff'd the candles, descended and delivered out to the company his hat-full of Syllabuses, divided into Sections No. 1, 2, 3, etc. (such stuff, and so printed, as to be entirely incoherent and unintelligible). Then mounting his scaffold, he bowed very low; then putting himself into a proper attitude, began, in a solemn, tragical voice and tone: "At Number 1 thus written you will find"—and repeating this with some vehemence, he read No. 1 of his Syllabus, speaking for two hours in the same manner, and with the same air, gesture, and tone, and making a sort of blank verse of it, and always ending with a verb—for that, he says, is the true Ciceronian, prodigiously difficult, and never attempted by any man in our language before. In some instances, he said, "He equal'd the finest periods Tully ever wrote or spoke"; which always began with the genitive case, were followed

* See p. 146. † Cafoy, a kind of fabric.

by the substantive, and concluded with the verb—as thus—"Of Th'
Eye, the Beauties I will now declare ——". This was often repeated,
as his masterpiece; and he exulted and admired himself vastly upon it.
When he had finished he came smiling among his Auditors, appealed
to them publicly if it was not charming fine, and if they had ever
heard anything like it. I must own I never did, or saw his equal; and
therefore send you this sketch of him as a great rarity.

The following incident also throws a small side-light on his
public appearances. In illustration of its marvellous powers he
used to undertake to express every human passion by the eye
alone. At Cambridge, one of his audience objected that there
was no merit in doing so when his hearers were told beforehand
what passion he was about to express; he demanded, therefore,
that they should be allowed to guess for themselves. "With all
my heart", said Taylor; "what do I look now?" "Why, pity,
I suppose." "Yes, you are quite right, sir", said the Chevalier;
and of course would have said the same had he guessed "rage"
or anything else ((63), 1781).

This somewhat crude method was no doubt sufficient to turn
the laugh against a hostile interrupter, but that he was really
capable of a smart repartee is shown by the following anec-
dote(99):

Taylor, the oculist, dining with the barristers upon the Oxford
circuit, having related many wonderful things which he represented
himself to have performed, was asked by Bearcroft, a little out of
humour with his self-conceit: "Pray, Chevalier, as you have told us
a great many things which you have done and can do, will you be so
good as to try to tell us anything which you cannot do?" "Nothing
so easy," replied Taylor, "I cannot pay my share of the dinner-bill,
and that, sir, I must beg of you to do."

The success of these methods was undoubtedly great.
Lecat(45) informs us that at Rouen, in 1743, the door of his
lodging was guarded by soldiers, that an introduction was
necessary to gain admission, and that he operated in the presence
of a brilliant circle of chosen persons. Rathlauw(52) states that in
1751 at Amsterdam, 170 persons sought Taylor's advice on the

day of his arrival, and that he himself only reached the great man with much trouble and cost. Curiously enough, the Chevalier's own estimate is more modest than these figures would seem to indicate. Writing in 1748, he says that for many years he had treated 1000 patients a year and sometimes more(29); with his usual indifference to matters of detail he probably did not pause to work out how many patients a day are signified by the resounding number, "a thousand".

Towards patients with means he is said, by hostile witnesses however, to have acted with shameless rapacity, demanding exorbitant fees for trifling services and threatening those who refused to pay with law-suits ((68), 1744). Eschenbach(38) states that he demanded (for operations presumably) 100 reichsthaler* from people of middle station, 100 to 300 ducats* from those in a better position, and 1000 ducats from the very rich; in one case he received 50 ducats a day for an ordinary cure. The statement of Stricker(96), that he received 500 ducats from the municipality of Amsterdam and 300 from that of the Hague, seems to be erroneous(100). On one occasion, when a patient with recurring inflammation of the eyes was brought to him, he immediately, and without being asked to do so, opened a vessel of the conjunctiva, and demanded 300 ducats(84). For an operation on a Danish apothecary named Günther, he received in advance a gold watch worth 100 ducats, and was promised 100 ducats in cash. The operation was a failure, Günther decamped without paying, and subsequently vexed the Chevalier with defamatory pamphlets(38, 88). In other cases also his expectations were disappointed. He bargained with Sir William Smyth for a fee of sixty guineas "if he restored his patient to any degree of sight". The operation was successful, and to the end of his life Sir William was able to read and write without the use of spectacles; he pretended, however, that his sight was exceedingly imperfect, and

* The reichsthaler or rixdollar varied in value from about 1s. 3d. to 4s. 9d. The gold ducat was worth about 9s. 5d.; the silver about half that amount (Webster's *Dictionary*).

finally drove Taylor to compound for twenty guineas(59). The Chevalier is not above relating tales of this kind against himself. When he looked for a fee, after curing a number of ladies in a convent, he was presented instead with an image of the Virgin, decked with flowers and inscribed with prayers; he had the good sense to accept the gift with becoming reverence. On another occasion, a rich man, instead of rewarding Taylor, gave a silver statue of himself to our Lady of Loretto(19). To the poor he was liberal in promises of free treatment, but he is said to have dismissed those who were really destitute, and to have squeezed unmercifully those who had something to pay(68).

TAYLOR AND THE MEDICAL PROFESSION

From an early period of his career the Chevalier's relations with the faculty began to be troubled. Even in Norwich days professional malice seized upon certain unsuccessful results at Yarmouth. Not content with aspersing his abilities, his persecutors, it seems, fell foul of his manners, holding that "if a man wore tolerable good Cloaths, and lik'd the Company of a Friend, 'twas impossible he could be a good Surgeon", and with regard to his discoveries that "if 'tis his own, 'twill not bear the light, if 'twill bear the light, 'tis not his own".

Yet it cannot be said that he was received at first with unreasoning hostility. In 1729, Benedict Duddell(37), the best English writer on ophthalmic subjects in the first half of the eighteenth century, wrote a work to correct certain errors in Taylor's *Mechanism of the Eye*. His tone is critical, but not hostile; he disagrees with Taylor's method of treating corneal nebulae and with his classification of opacities of the lens, draws attention to the importance of observing the mobility of the pupil before operating for cataract, and answers certain queries which Taylor had propounded. Later, however ((37 *a*), 1736), he gives an unfavourable account of the Chevalier's operating, saying that his hand shook, that vitreous was lost, and that his method of performing the operation for cataract did not correspond with his description.*

Probably about the year 1737 or 1738 a certain J.S., one of the "Surgeons of London and Westminster" to whom Taylor's book on cataract and glaucoma was dedicated, wrote a work entitled *Dr Taylor couched for a Cataract*(44). It is an exceedingly poor performance, with many cheap sneers and gibes, in which Taylor is accused of borrowing his knowledge from others and bungling their meaning with his jargon. The task of picking holes in the treatise on cataract was, perhaps, not a very difficult one, but when the author ventures to give his own views he falls into blunders worse than anything in the works of his antagonist.†
Stricker's(96) statement that Taylor left London on account of the publication of this pamphlet cannot surely be correct. I have been unable to trace another English polemic which is mentioned by Hirschberg(84), *A Receipt of a ready Composition on the Diseases of the . . . Eyes.*

On the Continent also the Chevalier's reception was mixed. He obtained favourable reports from Dr König, Professor of Theoretical Medicine in the University of Basel, and from Dr Gesner, of Zurich(2). The great Albrecht v. Haller referred to him as "a skilful man, but too liberal of promises"(40 a). The most judicial summing up of the Chevalier's claims, however, is found in a Latin oration delivered as a Rectorial Address, in 1750, by Professor Mauchart, of Tübingen(47). He first describes the

* Duddell seems to be the only author who impugns Taylor's operative skill. Mauchart (47), King (59), and Marteau (80), the last an eyewitness, give an opposite testimony. Taylor's grandson (97) was assured by Sir Walter Farquhar "that he was most sedulous in his attention, and that his manual dexterity appeared like the touch of magic. He may, indeed, be said to have been born with a genius for his art".

† As for the capsule of the lens, of which Taylor speaks, J.S. has never been able to see such a membrane; he tells us that when the four recti act together they shorten the axis of the eye, draw the lens *nearer* the retina, so that "we may see objects at a small distance more distinctly"; the obliqui, on the other hand, whose action is "more especially to be perceived in lovers and dying persons", elongate the eye and give clearer vision for distance. His explanation of the cause of cataract is certainly not more illuminating than Taylor's.

Chevalier's methods, as given in the last section, and recites his claim that his erudition, experience, affability, candour, and operative dexterity and promptitude are confirmed by public and private testimonies, and that in Amsterdam he failed to cure only fifteen out of 225 persons. On the other hand, objection has been made to his ostentation and histrionic tricks; it has been hinted that he bribes healthy persons to pretend a cure; specific instances of failure have been mentioned; it has been stated that his novelties are no novelties, or, if new, are puerilities. For his part Mauchart believes him to be a man well versed in the recognition of affections of the eye; instructed by ample experience and opportunities of observation; not destitute of ingenuity and judgment; striving genuinely to cultivate and adorn the difficult art of ophthalmology. In his treatises there is much that is candid and solid, even if some of it be not his own. Let him give up the practices which have brought him into ill-repute— his advertisements in public newspapers, his arrogance, his boasting. Let him collect his rare observations, enumerate his remedies, faithfully reveal his failures, and contract a friendship and literary commerce with other celebrated oculists. Especially let him give up his two claims (which move the saliva of the vulgar, the bile of the learned) that he can cure all cataracts and glaucomas without pain or danger, and that he has remedies for gutta serena and other diseases hitherto held incurable. His method of couching is not new nor the invention of Taylor, but was performed by Petit. As for gutta serena, how could it be cured if it were due, for instance, to destruction of the nerve by wound, atrophy, or compression? Mauchart does not deny, however, that some forms of gutta serena may be curable, and after all, the Chevalier's claim amounts to little more than this.

A favourable opinion, dating from the later career of the Chevalier, is contained in a letter of March 16th, 1765, addressed by Dr Marteau, of Amiens, to Petit(80). Marteau says that he has followed Taylor's practice for a month, and has seen him operate "d'une main aussi légère que sûre". He had imagined gutta serena to be a hopeless condition, but testifies to the cure of one case and the improvement of a second.

Among these favourable or semi-favourable estimates, however, are others of a more hostile cast. E. F. Heister(41), son of the better known Laurentius Heister, says that Taylor had little success in Amsterdam, rendered many people blind, and would have lost his following had he remained longer. Not one blind person, so far as he could learn, had been cured. Taylor was careful to secure his fee in advance, but had received letters from disappointed patients in Cologne demanding restitution. An instance of the disastrous results of his treatment is given (see p. 188).

Platner (1738, (50)) also alludes to the contempt with which prudent men must regard Taylor's pretentiousness, ostentation of learning, and inconsiderate temerity in treatment; by an affectation of ludicrous subtlety, and by boasting like a pedlar, that rash and notorious man, he says, has spread darkness rather than light over the discoveries of Petit and others.

Eschenbach(38), who saw something of Taylor's work when he was called to Rostock to treat the Duke of Mecklenburg-Schwerin, gives a dismal picture of his results. Not only was the treatment of the Duke a failure, but except for a few cases of senile cataract and slight ophthalmia no one else received any benefit. Some of his operative results were bad, and no case of gutta serena was cured. Eschenbach censures his blatant advertisements and mocks the growing numbers of his works, only one of which was written by himself—a statement in which the critic's temper has certainly got the better of his judgment.

A more personal note is struck in the delineations of two French authors, Caqué(80) and Lecat(45). Caqué met Taylor during his stay in Rheims in 1765.* He thought him an extraordinary man, and found him "très vif". Taylor spoke briefly in very bad French, which was difficult to understand; he explained his method of couching, which appeared to his visitor

* Given erroneously in the *Gaz. Méd. de Paris* as 1755.

to be a very reasonable operation. As he was taking his leave, however, Caqué learned with surprise that Taylor had been called to one of his patients, M. Favart, a Canon of the Cathedral, who had a cataract in each eye, complicated with central corneal ulcers. He resolved to take the opportunity of becoming acquainted with the Chevalier's methods, and therefore accompanied him to the Canon's house. Arrived there, Taylor took a little instrument of gold, fashioned like a file at its extremities, and passed it into the lower part of the conjunctival sac; he then closed this eye, applied a cold wet compress to both, secured it with a bandage of black taffeta which he drew from his pocket, and said to the patient "It is all over; you shall see to-morrow". He then opened the Canon's shirt collar, placed his thumb on one jugular while his assistant compressed the other, and with the greatest celerity bled the patient, "qui criait en m'appelant à son secours, ne sachant à quel saint se vouer". When Caqué reproached him with doing all this without giving the patient, or anyone else, warning of what he was about, he replied that he loved better to cure than to talk, and that when he did explain his intentions his patients usually became faint-hearted, or refused to have anything at all done.*

When Dr Caqué was subsequently asked his opinion of the Chevalier, his reply that he was "beaucoup plus charlatan qu'habile" will cause no surprise.

Lecat's account of the Chevalier is not less entertaining. Taylor, "cet homme spirituel, aimable", arrived in Rouen in 1765, and was the subject of general admiration. He had a superb arsenal of instruments and used them with dexterity; he showed innumerable laudatory and authentic testimonials. He visited Lecat several times, and finally took him to see his operations, promising to teach him his methods. Lecat scarcely quitted him for three days, and soon penetrated his pretences. His observations on Taylor's technique will be mentioned later. The

* Perhaps this explanation accounts for his treatment of the patient with recurring inflammation, mentioned on p. 150.

Chevalier had mentioned a certain nerve which he divided in his operation for squint, and had promised to show it to Lecat at the first opportunity. The latter, therefore, procured a human head, dissected it carefully, and proved the absence of any such filament. Being seated at dinner with Taylor on the same day, he easily turned the conversation once more to the nervous filament, and again obtained the promise of a demonstration. A covered dish was brought in, the cover was removed, and there lay the dissected human head; to a connoisseur it would have been an object of interest; to Taylor it was "une vraie tête de Méduse". He sat petrified, while Lecat favoured him with a *critique raisonnée* of his pretensions, and adjured him to use with honesty the happy talents with which nature had endowed him. In a few days Taylor's vogue was past, the squints and corneal opacities which he had operated on were as before, and most of his cataract cases were blind.

Guérin(39), another French surgeon, writing in 1770, gives an equally unfavourable account. Taylor had an operation for every disease of the eye, his sole object being to obtain prompt, if illusive, cures. He used all the most refined devices of charlatanism and deceit to dupe those whom his reputation brought within his clutches. When he had performed an operation "il chantoit victoire, il crioit au miracle", he then bandaged the eye, with a strict injunction not to uncover it for five or six days, but, having levied his spoils, he himself decamped on the fourth.

There are instances also in which the profession took corporate action to expose the practices of the quack. In 1744, glowing accounts having appeared in the Edinburgh newspapers of Taylor's knowledge, success and charity, the Incorporation of Surgeons published an advertisement, giving the opposite side of the picture. This stimulated a certain Dr George Young to take up the cudgels in his behalf. Taylor's skill in treatment and his dexterity in operating, founded on a vast experience, exceeded anything which Young had ever seen; his persecution was due to his having succeeded in some cases where the regular faculty had failed. On this the Royal College of Physicians issued a declaration, stating that Taylor had inserted in the newspapers advertisements "stuffed with gross, injurious falsehoods", such as that his lectures were constantly attended by the chief members of the Faculty of the University, and that his methods were approved by the most eminent of the profession. In point of fact no professor had been present at a single lecture. Curiosity, indeed, had attracted individual members, who had reported that his lectures were trifling; that his operations were attended with very indifferent success; that the health of many of his patients had been impaired by excessive and unnecessary evacuations and other irregular methods of practice; that in difficult cases he had proposed absurd and destructive methods of cure, and when opposed by regular physicians had proclaimed that he was hindered from completing the cure;* that he had undertaken incurable cases, and demanded exorbitant fees even from those in low circumstances; and that his promises of gratuitous treatment were merely a fraudulent device ((68), 1744).

After this it is a little surprising to find the Chevalier dedicating one of his books(9) to the President and Fellows of the Royal College of Physicians at Edinburgh, in the following terms:

"The grateful Remembrance I have, of the Attention which some of your Body judged me worthy of, by so frequently favouring me with their Presence at my Lectures, and Method of Practice, and by their giving me such undeniable Proofs of the good Opinion they have of me, from the many they have recommended to my Care, encourage me to believe, etc., etc."

In Amsterdam also the Professors of Anatomy and Surgery, Inspectors of the Medical College, and Physicians of the City addressed a circular in Dutch and French to the principal journals (1749), stating that Taylor's announcements were false, and that the results of his treatment on a previous visit fifteen years before had been disastrous(100).

* This is the Chevalier's plea in *The Case of Sir Jeremy Sambrooke* (22).

In replying to these attacks Taylor was at first inclined to be abusive. He told his persecutors that their gravity was natural dullness, and that "an Awkward Saint-like Behaviour, a Solemn Gait, an Hypocritical Elevation of the Eye, and an affected Religious Grimace, is sufficient with them to set a Man at the Head of his Profession". But he was too clever not to perceive very soon that injured innocence was a far better cue. In his later works he poses as a sadly misunderstood man; himself fully qualified, he cannot understand why the profession should be against him; he has never refused to consult with them, nor appropriated their patients(19); he has nothing but kindly feelings towards his brethren; and has always been treated with the greatest respect by those who have really known him(29); it was only the hope of earning their approbation that made him undertake so many toilsome journeys(2); in his book on Cataract and Glaucoma(3) he recommends that the after-treatment of operation cases should be carried out with the assistance of a physician. The very name of quackery arouses in him a generous indignation. England is much too lenient in this matter. It is a pity the laws as to examinations are not more strictly enforced. Abroad unqualified practice is criminal; he has met many quack oculists and seen them banished and imprisoned, but needless to say has never himself been molested.

Pursuing the same line of tactics, it was his custom when he arrived in any town to make himself known to the learned, and, as we have seen, to invite them to his lectures. A similar device was to dedicate his books to the most eminent members of the profession, or in more general terms to the "Physicians and Surgeons of London and Westminster", "Messieurs de l'Académie des Sciences", "The President and Fellows of the Royal College of Physicians at Edinburgh, etc."

The defence of ophthalmology as a specialism is a favourite theme with the Chevalier. So difficult an art demands the devotion of a lifetime, yet, on the other hand, it can only be practised in a rational manner by one who has a thorough knowledge of the human economy, acquired by a regular course of study. Such a man is Taylor himself, and he is the first example of an oculist who has been also a physician.

TAYLOR IN THE EYES OF LAY CONTEMPORARIES

References to Taylor in the classical literature of the eighteenth century are scanty. The passing allusion of Gibbon(56) has been mentioned (p. 139). Horace Walpole(61) warns a friend against his practices in these terms: "I need not desire you not to believe the stories of such a mountebank as Taylor; I only wonder that he should think the names of our family a recommendation at Rome; we are not conscious of any such merit; nor have any of our eyes ever wanted to be put out". He also wrote an extremely poor epigram founded on the title *Chevalier* de St George assumed by the Old *Pretender*:

> Why Taylor the quack calls himself *Chevalier*
> 'Tis not easy a reason to render;
> Unless blinding eyes, that he thinks to make clear,
> Demonstrates he's but a *Pretender*.

In *The Ghost* Churchill(55) refers to him as follows:

> But if (for it is our intent
> Fairly to state the argument)
> A Man should want an eye or two,
> The Remedy is sure, tho' new;
> The Cure's at hand—no need to fear—
> For proof—behold the *Chevalier*—
> As well prepar'd, beyond all doubt,
> To put Eyes in as put them out.

A more favourable impression may be gathered from the following sketch by Dr William King, Principal of St Mary's Hall, Oxford(59); the story of how his grandfather, Sir William Smyth, cheated the Chevalier has already been related (p. 151).

I was at Tunbridge in 1748, where I met with the Chevalier Taylor, the famous oculist. He seems to understand the anatomy of the eye perfectly well; he has a fine hand and good instruments, and performs all his operations with great dexterity; for the rest, *Ellum homo fidens*; who undertakes anything (even impossible cases) and promises everything. No charlatan ever appeared with fitter and more excellent talents or to a greater advantage; he has a good person, is a natural orator, and has a facility of learning foreign languages.* He has travelled over all Europe, and always with an equipage suitable to a man of the first quality, and hath been introduced to most of the sovereign princes, from whom he has received many marks of their liberality and esteem—titles, orders, medals, rings, pictures, etc. He is an honorary member of many foreign universities, and has published his works in Latin, English, French, Spanish, and Italian. He pretends to know the secrets of all courts, and to be as skilful a politician as he is an oculist. He returned to England, as he told me, in hopes of being immediately introduced to his Majesty (George II), and recommended as the only person able to cure the King's eyes; but he has not hitherto succeeded in this attempt, nor in other respects been so highly considered by his own countrymen as by foreign nations. The following character,† which I had drawn of him, he entreated me to publish, as what he conceived would do him honour.

Another "character", also in the form of a Latin Elogium, and probably by the same hand, will be found in the Bodleian Library (see Appendix IV).

A character so frothy as Taylor's was little likely to commend itself to the solid common-sense of Dr Johnson. His verdict according to Boswell(54) was as follows:

"Taylor was the most ignorant man I ever knew; but sprightly. Ward the dullest.‡ Taylor challenged me once to talk Latin with him (laughing). I quoted some of Horace, which he took to be part of my own speech. He said a few words well enough". Beauclerk: "I remember, Sir, you said that Taylor was an instance how far impudence could carry ignorance".

* For a different view concerning his oratory see the letter of Palmer (p. 148); concerning his facility in learning languages, the opinion of Caqué (p. 155).

† See Appendix (p. 212).

‡ Steevens also says, "I was assured by the late Dr Johnson that Ward was the weakest and Taylor the most ignorant of the whole empiric tribe". A critic in a contemporary journal summed him up as "a coxcomb, but a coxcomb of parts" (97).

It should be said, however, that by "ignorant" Johnson probably meant ignorant of scholarship, and especially of classical learning. It is true that in one of his innumerable poses the Chevalier portrays himself as a profound Latinist, and laments that there is no law against translating the language of science into the vulgar tongue; and he adorns one of his dedications(34) with a plethora of Latin tags, which he condescends to translate for the benefit of the uninitiated. But with these exceptions he seldom lays much claim to that particular type of knowledge. His books, on the other hand, testify that he was a man of some education, and possessed a considerable, if not always perfectly grammatical, command of the English language.

Apart from these graver estimates, it was to be expected that the Chevalier's striking personality should attract a shower of pasquinades, lampoons, and squibs of all kinds. As it happens, we possess examples of the wit of London, Edinburgh and Dublin. London's contribution is a "ballad opera", called *The Operator*(73), in which Taylor figures as "Dr Hurry, an oculist".

One of the scenes represents a hall in the doctor's house. The assembled patients have heard that he does not take money, but it is rumoured that there is a secretary who "holds out the palm". The doctor, they are informed, has thirteen lords and dukes with him that morning. Presently he enters; there is a general distribution of snuff, which, he assures them, is a panacea for all diseases. When the people remind him of his advertisements of free treatment he replies that the fees which he exacts are to supply remedies for the poor. To one woman who says she has nothing, he answers that it makes no difference at all, but he happens to be exceedingly busy that morning. He tells some medical men who visit him that he can cure gutta serena "with one drop of my collyrium", and confesses that he "purchased a diploma for gold at Padua". Asked his opinion of Sir William Read (another famous quack, oculist to Queen Anne), he calls him a "mere nurse, a mere washer-woman, in respect of what I do". He quotes, with approval, the father's advice: "Get money honestly, son, if you can; however, get money".* He admits that

* "Get money, money—fairly if you may,
    If not, be sure you get it any way."   *Horace*, Epist. I, i. Transl. Theod. Martin.

when he began to practise he blinded 300 people.* A supposed blind man is brought in, and Dr Hurry is adjured to tell the truth for once; he promises to do so—there is no hope. It turns out that the man sees perfectly. In the last scene the doctor treats all his duns and creditors at a tavern, and then decamps, leaving them to pay the bill, whereupon the pawnbroker consoles the others with the following couplet:

"But let us be gay, and our losses despise,
And rejoice that we've safely escap'd with our eyes".

The Edinburgh lampoon is entitled *A Faithful and Full Account of the Surprising Life and Adventures of the Celebrated Doctor Sartorius Sinegradibus*(70). It is a mere extravaganza relating the prodigies which preceded the birth of the great man; how he began to read anatomy, physic, optics and surgery, but, finding the process laborious, burnt his books, collected a quantity of aqueous, vitreous and crystalline humours, and drank them off, at the same time bleeding himself at the temporal artery and jugular vein, so as to draw off the gross blood and fill his head with purer juices; how, employing himself exclusively with vision, he shut off all his other senses by putting corks in his ears, etc.; how he fell into an illness, but was cured when money was clinked before him—and so forth. Some mock testimonials are added—if the eyes are weak and tender the doctor will so manage that the strongest light shall not affect them—he makes one-eyed persons see with both alike, etc.

The title of the Dublin book is *The English Impostor detected; or, the History of the Life and Fumigation of the Renown'd Mr J— T—, Oculist*(69). It is a work without merit, written in a mock heroic style, and giving an account of an unsavoury practical joke played upon Taylor by some young men of Dublin.

The publication in 1761 of Taylor's *Travels and Adventures* produced a burlesque imitation, *The Life and extraordinary History of the Chevalier John Taylor*, purporting to be written by his son(71). Fortunately, however, the son's reputation can be

---

* I do not know whether there is any other foundation than this passage for the statement in Hirschberg, p. 296 (84), that Taylor himself "jestingly" confessed to having blinded 300 Swiss.

cleared from the impiety of having so grossly traduced his father. The book is introduced by a supposed letter from the Chevalier, to which the son replies that he has "maintained my mother these eight Years, and do at this present Time; and that two Years since, I was concerned in his Affairs, for which I have paid near £200". It can be shown, however, that the two were on good terms at this period; in the authentic *Travels and Adventures* the Chevalier praises his son's abilities, supports a proposal of his to found an institution for treating "the numberless distressed blind", and promises to give his own assistance in carrying out the project.

The account of the whole matter given by Taylor's grandson(97) is as follows: After the publication of his memoirs the Chevalier went abroad, and not long afterwards a report of his death reached England. His son thereupon formed the project of publishing a plain, unvarnished account of Taylor's life, "wholly free from that egotism which certainly characterised the Chevalier's own biography", and even entered into negotiations with Dodsley, the publisher, to that end. But finding himself unversed in literary pursuits, he submitted his materials to Henry Jones, a disreputable Irish poet and dramatist, who lost them during an unavoidable midnight change of lodgings. A public announcement of the intended work and of Jones's participation was, however, already in circulation, and that "profligate scribbler", who had been paid in advance, had the impudence to bring out his ribald version, partly from his recollection of the lost notes, but chiefly from the resources of his own malicious invention. The work was repudiated, but apparently the author was not considered worth the powder and shot of legal proceedings.

As for the book itself, it is a mere tissue of scandalously indecent incidents in the worst style of eighteenth-century licentiousness, and without the least atom of credibility. Its only interest is derived from some confirmation which it affords of Taylor's having studied under Cheselden at St Thomas's, and of the honours which he received in Portugal; it also bears an enemy's testimony to his personal fascination—"for bating a little of the Knight Errant—there was something whimsical and not disagreeable mixed with his manner".

In addition to these more elaborate skits, a number of satirical references may be found in the newspapers of the time. In these Taylor is frequently associated with two other famous quacks— Mrs Mapp, sometimes known as Crazy Sally, a bone-setter, and Ward (mentioned, as stated above, by Johnson and Gibbon), the inventor of Ward's pill, to which there is frequent allusion in eighteenth-century literature. In the *Gentleman's Magazine*(63) for October 16th, 1736, for instance, we read what is presumably not to be regarded as a strictly authentic piece of news.

Mrs Mapp the Bone-setter, with Dr Taylor, the Oculist, being at the Playhouse in Lincoln's Inn Fields, to see a Comedy call'd the "Husband's Relief", with the Female Bone-setter and Worm Doctor, it occasion'd a full house, and the following epigram:

"While Mapp to the actors show'd a kind regard,
On one side Taylor sat, on th' other Ward;
When their mock persons of the Drama came,
Both Ward and Taylor thought it hurt their Fame;
Wondr'd how Mapp could in good humour be,
Zoons crys the Manly Dame, it hurts not me;
Quacks without Art may either blind or kill;
But Demonstration shows that mine is Skill".*

Another poem of 1736(86) begins:

Of late without the least pretence to skill
Ward's grown a famed physician by a pill.

And goes on:

Next travell'd Taylor fill'd us with surprise,
Who pours new light upon the blindest eyes;
Each journal tells his circuit through the land;
Each journal tells the blessing of his hand:
And, lest some hireling scribbler of the town
Injures his history, he writes his own.
We read the long account with wonder o'er;
Had he wrote less we had believ'd him more.

* This alludes to some cures she is said to have performed before Sir Hans Sloane at the Grecian Coffee House.

And yet another tells us:

> Forgot is the bustle 'bout Taylor and Ward;
> Now Mapp's all the cry, and her fame's on record.

The following is taken from the *Daily Journal*, of November 16th, 1736:

> Three famous Quacks in one country born,
> Epsom, Pallmall and Suffolk-street adorn:
> M—p makes the Lame to walk by manuel slight;
> T—r alike restores the Blind to Sight,
> The Stone, the Gout, the P—x, and every ill
> W—d cures internally by Drop and Pill.
> Ye Quacks in Medicine prescribe no more;
> Without it, these, as sure as Death, can cure.

In the *St James's Evening Post*, of July 19th, 1737, there is an announcement that, "This day was published, beautifully printed price 6*d*., 'An Epistle to a Young Student at Cambridge; with the Characters of the three great Quacks, Mapp, Taylor, and Ward: with the methods they used to make themselves famous'" I have been unable to obtain a perusal of this pamphlet.

The three associates had the honour of being painted in 1736 by Hogarth in his *Consultation of Physicians*(86). They are placed in a gallery above the twelve physicians who crowd the foreground of the picture. In the centre is Mrs Mapp holding a bone; on one side Taylor leans upon her with one eye closed in a leer; in the head of his cane an eye is depicted; on the opposite side is Ward, with half his face darkened to represent a mole, which earned him the name of "Spot" Ward.

In the *Scots Magazine* of 1744 (p. 32), there is a Latin poem comparing Taylor with George Whitfield, the Methodist preacher, of all people! Both alike are most illustrious mountebanks, one a tailor of eyes (*oculorum sartor*), the other a corrupter of souls; befogging one the bodily, the other the mental vision; both destroyers of our fatherland, etc. (see Appendix V, p. 214). A semi-political, satirical Latin epistle to the Chevalier, not over-remarkable for wit, will be found in the *Gentleman's Magazine* of 1736, p. 647 (see Appendix VI, p. 215).

Lastly, mention may be made of a broadsheet ballad in the British Museum, which relates a quarrel between Taylor and some member of the profession who had refused him the use of his infirmary—in what town is not stated (see Appendix VII, p. 217).

TAYLOR'S WORKS

Taylor's works are said to have been published in Latin, English, French, German, Italian, Spanish, Portuguese, Danish, Swedish and Russian; in fact, books are still extant in the first five of these languages. That he employed translators goes without saying, and unquestionably he must have received help in some of his dedications, but there is no reason to doubt that the main body of his works is his own. A similarity of style runs through them, and the same views and opinions, even on minor matters, recur in books published at widely separate periods.

In these works we find two voices, the voice of the mountebank and the voice of the man of sense and observation. Of the former let the following suffice(19). I condense considerably:

O! thou mighty; oh! thou sovereign pontiff; oh! thou great luminary of the church; given to mankind . . . as a star to the Christian world. . . . Who can believe, that you, most holy father, who art placed as the first inspector of the deeds of man, would proclaim to all the inhabitants of the earth, as you have done, your high approbation of my works but by the voice of truth?

Oh! ye imperial; oh! ye royal; oh! ye great masters of empire; who have so far extended your benevolence as to be witnesses of my labours. . . . How often have you condescended to behold the transports that affected the mind, when from before the dark eye, by my hands, the dismal veil was removed, the curtain drawn; and saw, by my labours, this beauteous little globe re-assume its native power, and was again a lucid orb! Who then can suppose that you . . . would point out, as it were with the sceptre in hand, me alone amongst all mankind for these things, but from the strongest evidence that could be possibly desired for the support of truth?

Oh! ye empresses; oh! ye queens: ... you whose gentleness, whose goodness of heart, have so often engaged your awful presence on these occasions—what satisfaction have you expressed at seeing the blind, by me, enabled to behold again the marvels of heaven! And finding them prostrate at your feet, expressing their joy at what they first saw; because 'twas you they saw—the first object of their duty—the highest in their wishes, etc.

If this kind of bombast represented the Chevalier's contributions to literature they would little repay study; but in fact it is confined, for the most part, to his dedications and prefatory letters, and to the *Travels and Adventures*. In this respect a comparison of his earlier with his later works reveals something of a Rake's Progress. The *Mechanism of the Eye* (1727) is remarkably free from immoderate claims. He acknowledges that he is wholly indebted to Cheselden for the "knowledge I have of this Branch of my Profession, such as it is", and that he received his first hint as to the treatment of cataract from the same source; he tells us that he does not "propose to give any new Theory of Vision, nor to be able to describe the manner of it better than it is already done by an eminent Author";* he admits failure, and expresses his obligation "to a very ingenious Gentleman . . . for Two or Three Hints that he has given me". Before long, however, the cloven hoof begins to appear. Already, in 1736(3), he informs us that "nothing . . . has yet appeared in our Language worth the least notice" on the subject of which he treats, and from this date onwards his dedications usually consist of nothing but a string of impertinences.

In the body of his works, however, Taylor usually drops his posturing and writes plain English. It is to be understood, of course, that not all the facts and methods analysed in the following pages are original discoveries of his own. Some real contributions to ophthalmic knowledge he did make, but all that can fairly be expected of a writer of general treatises, such as form the majority of Taylor's works, is a sound knowledge of

* Berkeley, whose *New Theory of Vision* was published in 1709.

his subject, a judicious selection of his facts, some originality in commenting upon them in the light of his own experience, and a sprinkling of original observations. These qualities are not lacking in Taylor's best works, and, leaving aside the question of originality, a *résumé* of his opinions may be justified, on general historical grounds, by the insight which it affords into the workings of a shrewd eighteenth-century mind on the problems of ophthalmic science.

PHYSIOLOGY

Taylor's description of the anatomy of the eye calls for no special remark; it is a sufficiently accurate compendium of contemporary knowledge. His views on the more elusive subject of physiology are of greater interest.

Optics, Refraction, Binocular Vision. The account of the optics and refraction of the eye which is given in the *Mechanismus* (4 *a*) is in the main correct, and is illustrated by good diagrams. Emmetropia, hypermetropia, myopia, and the correction of errors of refraction by means of convex and concave glasses are accurately described. Hypermetropia and myopia are due to an insufficient or too great convexity of the cornea, which also becomes flatter with increasing age. Those who are perplexed by the fact that the inverted image on the retina is seen upright, should reflect that behind the retina there is no second invisible eye which beholds the image. It is the mind which performs the rectification. He is indebted to Bishop Berkeley for some of these ideas, and, indeed, quotes that writer's *Alciphron, or the Minute Philosopher* ((4 *a*), p. 173), but not the fuller account of the same subject in the *New Theory of Vision.*

On the reason why we see singly with two eyes Taylor's remarks could scarcely be bettered. The crossing at the chiasma is correctly described, and the connexion of the two retinae with the nerve-centres is neatly illustrated by a comparison with a bell whose single rope (the optic tract) has two ends (half of each optic nerve); a pull on either or both of the ends will ring the bell. Corresponding points and the diplopia induced by artificial displacement of the globe are well known to him. The optic nerves necessarily enter on one side of the posterior pole; otherwise the two blind spots, being corresponding points, central vision would be obliterated; they necessarily enter on the nasal side, because the image of a single object may be formed on the two temporal retinae, but cannot be formed on the two nasal retinae. Binocular vision is useful in the judgment of distance, but is not absolutely essential to it; after the loss of one eye the estimation is difficult, but it can be re-acquired by practice.

Regarding accommodation Taylor's first thoughts were better than his second. He tells us(1) that the power of seeing objects at different distances "is very probably lodg'd in the crystalline humour; which, according to the different distances of objects, approaches nigher to, or removes further from the retina, and *perhaps too assumes a different convexity*".* He notes that after a cataract operation objects are held at a greater distance.

Subsequently, however, in consequence of an erroneous observation that accommodation is preserved after couching, he abandoned the idea that changes in the form of the lens furnished the whole explanation. He still believed that the lens changed its position, and he discusses the opinion of those who hold that the ciliary ligament is a muscle which displaces the lens forward, either directly or by compressing the vitreous. He rejects this view, however, because if the ciliary ligament were a muscle vision should be clear for two distances only—when the muscle is contracted and when it is relaxed—and also because this mechanism would not account for the accommodation after couching. The displacement of the lens, he finally concludes, is due to the pressure of the external muscles, which causes also an elongation of the globe and an increased convexity of the cornea; normal accommodation depends on these three factors, and accommodation after couching on the second and third(4).

* According to Hirschberg this was first stated by Pemberton in 1719.

Pupil. The reaction of the pupil to light and on viewing near objects, Taylor says, is an involuntary act, but he has known persons who could induce the movement voluntarily by imagining an object in the air(4). On the other hand, some persons can see at various distances without the occurrence of any movement of the pupil. He has seen persons with very small and immobile pupils who yet saw well. His knowledge of the consensual reaction of the pupil may have been derived from Boerhaave, who is said to have first described it in 1708 (Hirschberg). The observation was made on a patient who had lost the sight of one eye after a fever. "In this case", he says, "it is remarkable, that when both eyes are exposed to Light, the Pupil of the diseas'd Eye maintains the same Changes with regard to its Change of Diameter, *i.e.*, to the Velocity of these Changes ∴ as the Pupil of the healthful Eye; and that on closing the well Eye, the Pupil of the diseased Eye. . . dilates slowly to near twice its Diameter, and continues immobile in that dilated State in all Degrees of Light, till the healthful Eye is again exposed to Light, when it contracts" ((9), p. 172).

Somewhat unexpected also is his knowledge of the significance of an association of mobile pupils with blindness. The condition occurs in two forms, one due to dropsy, the other to loss of blood. In the former the visual defect "is not for Want of the Nerves maintaining their healthful Perfection, but proceeds from the Brain's being in a State incapable of receiving the Idea of such Impression". After loss of blood the cerebral functions are also defective. The lesion is probably "in or about the Origin of the Nerves of the immediate organ of Sight".

Physiology of Vision. The most complete account of Taylor's views on the physiology of vision is contained in his *Impartial Inquiry into the Seat of the Immediate Organ of Sight*, published in 1743(7). In spite of its erroneous conclusion that the choroid is the visual organ, this work, by its freedom from bombast, judicious marshalling of the facts on both sides, close argument, and evidence of a wide knowledge of contemporary problems, conveys a more favourable impression than perhaps any other of its author's writings. His line of argument in support of the above conclusion may be summarised as follows:

(1) When sight is lost, the pupil becomes immobile. Therefore, there must be a connexion between the nerves of sight and those controlling the pupil. Now it is evident that the nerves of the choroid extend forward into the iris, but there is no such extension of the retina. The retina, therefore, cannot be the organ of sight. Against this reasoning, however, it might be argued that the movements of the pupil are not absolutely essential to vision. It is sometimes immobile although the patient sees well, and, on the other hand, good vision may be obtained through an artificial pupil, or through a number of openings in the iris, a condition which he has known to follow small-pox. Moreover, the opposite condition occurs, mobile pupils with blindness, but such cases are of cerebral origin and do not concern the present enquiry. The partisans of the retina also maintain that since the optic nerve and the nerves of the iris are all contained within the dura (it was thought that nerves were continued forward from the pia into the choroid), it may well be impossible to have one affected without the other.

(2) A connexion between the nerves of the iris and those of the visual organ is also proved by the fact that in many diseases exposure to light is painful, and in these diseases the pupil is always smaller than in the other eye. Sudden exposure to a brilliant light causes pain and a contraction of the pupil.

(3) It may be argued that the choroid, which is relatively poor in nerves, is less likely than the retina, which is an expansion of the optic nerve, to be the seat of vision. But the organ of vision need not be nervous in all its parts. The retina itself contains vessels, so that after all the difference is merely one of degree; nor have we any means of judging to what extent a nervous structure is necessary to vision; if the choroidal nerves are capable of moving the iris, why should they not be sufficient for the act of seeing? As regards the claim of the retina, it is known that the entrance of the optic nerve is blind; is it not probable, therefore, that its expansion is also blind? Moreover, wounding of the retina during an operation is followed by no ill consequences, whereas wounding of the long ciliary nerves (according to a firm conviction of Taylor's) necessarily entails blindness; it is worth considering also "whether the insensibility of the brain observable on

wounding it, be not a proof of the insensibility of the optic nerve, and consequently of its expansion, the retina".

(4) The living retina is too transparent to be the organ of vision. It is not the glass but the silvering on the back which receives the image. At any rate, it is extremely unlikely, that the membrane should both receive impressions and at the same time transmit sufficient light to the choroid to stimulate the choroidal nerves and cause contraction of the pupil. (It will be understood that this was the only mechanism of the pupillary movement likely to suggest itself to an eighteenth-century observer, ignorant, as he necessarily was, of the nature of reflex action.)

(5) Certain animals have brilliant colours in their choroids, and these animals have weaker sight; they see better in the dark, but endure more pain in a bright light than man. The anatomical difference resides in the choroid, not in the retina; and so also must the physiological. It has been argued, however, and is possible, that "the retina is, by the reflection of the Light striking on this Colour of the Choroides, made more sensible of the Impression of Objects". It may also be argued that the black colour of the choroid in man will render it unsuitable for the reception of images, black having the quality of absorbing rays of light.

(6) Some not very lucid proofs are adduced from the supposed nature of muscae volitantes. Taylor had a firm belief, elaborated more at length in his *Maladies de l'Organe immédiat de la Vûë* (2), that muscae are due to distension of the retinal arteries, preventing light from falling on the immediate organ of vision. If the retina were the immediate organ this distension would compress the nervous elements and prevent the patient from seeing objects clearly, as those subject to muscae frequently do.

(7) An argument against the choroid is the connexion of one retina with the other by means of the decussation of the optic nerves, an arrangement which must have something to do with binocular vision. To this objection no efficient reply is made.

If, then, the choroid is the immediate organ of sight, of what use is the retina? Its function is "to modify the Rays of Light in such a Manner, as that they shall not pass with too much Violence, for the Perfection of Vision". It is to the choroid what the epidermis is to the inner skin, and it is the inner skin, not the epidermis, which is the seat of sensation. On the other hand, if the retina should turn out to be the seat of vision the function of the choroid is probably the absorption of the superfluous rays of light.

CATARACT

In Taylor's early days the echoes of the controversy as to the true seat of cataract had not completely died away. The opinion of Brisseaux and Maître Jan, that cataract was an affection of the lens was, no doubt, generally accepted, but whether membranous cataracts also existed was still a matter of argument. The discussion was in some degree academic—whether or not inflammatory membranes in the pupil should be *called* cataracts—but, at any rate, we find Taylor on the right side of the controversy. He marshals the arguments for and against the two views, quotes his authorities, refers to the dissections of Petit, admits that pupillary membranes do occur, but maintains that they are not cataracts, and cannot be couched(3).

His views on causation are not very illuminating. The affection may follow a blow, violent grief, or the unskilful treatment of an ophthalmia if the discharge, instead of being "allured forwards by kind Discutients", is "drove back by cold Repellents". The actual cause of the opacity is a viscidity of the blood, so that nourishment is separated in too small quantity, or the nourishing particles have a figure or magnitude not adapted to pass through the pores of the lens(1). He afterwards developed a theory that the condition was due to the pressure of the external muscles on the globe, and was, therefore, caused by "a long constant Direction of the Eye to particular Objects"(3). At one time he had a fantastic idea that the age of a cataract might be determined "by a Gradation of Colouring settled from Sir Isaac Newton's Theory, beginning at a light Blue and ending at a greenish Yellow"(1).

Of more importance are his views on the practical question, what cataracts should be operated on. He recognised that milky cataracts were dangerous, but he knew no way of judging their consistence before operation. He advises that unilateral cataracts should be left alone, because the operation "may be the occasion of the loss of both eyes". There can be no doubt that in his early days he was ignorant of the means of diagnosing amaurosis in a cataractous eye ((1), p. 64), but in later life he seems to have recognised clearly enough the importance of observing the pupil reaction. In this, as in many other instances, however, his cupidity overcame his better knowledge, and in his later works he vaunts his "new method of removing cataracts at all times, and in every species, without any Inflammation, or the Possibility of an Accident", and claims to be the first "to avoid that painful Delay of a Cataract's maturity"(3).

The operation described in Taylor's earliest work ((1), 1727) is an ordinary couching; in his treatise on Cataract and Glaucoma ((3), 1736) he elaborates a much more complicated procedure. His exposition is exceedingly involved, perhaps intentionally so, but with attentive reading the main steps, and the reasons for them, are sufficiently plain. At first he used no speculum, having "seen so many Inconveniences attend the Use of the Common *Speculum Oculi*; that . . . I have chose to have nothing to assist me, except the Pressure of the Thumb and Finger"; he soon began to use one, however(37), and subsequently claims to have invented "An instrument that has the Power to fix the Axes of both Eyes, the fixing one rendering the other on which he operates immoveable"(29).

A scleral incision was first made with a lancet in a downward and outward direction, a line and a half from the limbus and two lines below the horizontal meridian. A plano-convex needle—why it had this form is not very clear—was then passed through the incision to the lower equator of the lens, and the lens having been moved a little to see that the needle was properly placed, the capsule was opened below. The lower anterior part of the vitreous was now broken up a little with the needle in order to prepare a place for the lens, and so prevent it from rising again. The needle was then carried to the upper equator, where pressure was made so as to cause the lens substance to be extruded through the opening in the capsule below, into the place prepared for it in the vitreous. The rising of the lens was also to be prevented by evacuating certain watery humours which it contained, thus making it heavier than the vitreous.

The idea underlying these steps was to leave the upper part of the capsule and suspensory ligament intact; the vitreous bulging forward would therefore push the posterior against the anterior capsule and would mould itself on the apposed layers so as to take the shape of the absent lens and give vision nearly as good as in the normal eye. Moreover, "if we believe that the *Ligamentum Ciliare* (*i.e.* suspensory ligament) is in any manner necessary to our seeing Objects at different distances, whether from altering the Figure or changing the Situations of the Chrystalline; such Uses of it are very nearly preserved after this Operation".

Immediately after the operation a mixture of tincture of Peruvian balsam and warm water was dropped into the eye for some minutes, and a cataplasm of the same mixture with pulp of cassia was applied. On the second morning the eye was fomented with "a spirituous Fomentation with Camphire", and the bandage was replaced by a shade. Light diet and gentle evacuations were continued for twenty days. As a rule, apparently, he did not prescribe cataract glasses; no doubt he had usually resumed his peregrinations before his patients were ready for them, and in any case, as has been seen, he held that couching did not entail the loss of accommodation, and that his method of operating produced but little alteration in the refraction of the eye. Yet in early days he tells us that "if the Subjects I have hitherto performed the Operation upon were of Consideration enough to have given me Pains beyond my Needle, I make no Doubt, but I could have fixed them with Glasses which would have . . . made them some Amends for the loss of the aforesaid Humour"(1).

The main features of this operation—the opening of the capsule below and the pressing out of the lens substance through the aperture—are the invention of Petit.* The preliminary incision with the lancet, the use of the blunt needle, the preparing of a place in the vitreous, the alleged evacuation of fluid from the lens, and perhaps some of the theoretical considerations, appear to be contributions of more than doubtful value, added by Taylor.

To us it seems evident that such an operation could not be performed without rupturing the suspensory ligament. Did Taylor really attempt it, or is his elaborate description merely a charlatan device to impress the credulous? Lecat ((45), 1743) informs us that in spite of his assertions he really operated like anyone else, using Cheselden's needle, which he claimed as an invention of his own. On the other hand, Duddell's account ((37), 1735) corresponds more nearly with the operation mentioned above than with an ordinary couching, though he states that Taylor's performance did not correspond with his description; he says that a scleral incision three lines long was made with a lancet, and that a thick blunt needle was introduced. One might infer perhaps that in 1736, the year of publication of the treatise on Cataract and Glaucoma, Taylor was attempting the special operation, but that he afterwards gave it up for couching by the ordinary method; and, in fact, in 1749 we find him singing the praises of a new needle which was "round and very small" (68). But in 1765 Marteau (80)—a witness of somewhat facile belief, it is true—who had followed his operations for a month, again describes the scleral incision, the opening of the capsule below, and the preparation of the place in the vitreous; and informs us that at this stage of the operation a blunt needle of gold was substituted to perform the final depression.

There seems to be no doubt, therefore, that Taylor really did attempt this method, though perhaps not continuously throughout his career. If the main idea was Petit's, then evidently Taylor's reputation is cleared from the imputation of a charlatan invention, and his knowledge of the work of others is vindicated.

* *Hist. de l'Acad. Royale des Sciences*, 1725, 7e février, pp. 6–20.

Was the operation of extraction ever performed by Taylor? It has been stated that he first gave Daviel the idea of becoming an oculist(90), and a claim for priority in the extraction operation itself has even been advanced on his behalf. Both these statements are erroneous, however. The two men cannot have met before 1734, when Taylor was in Marseilles, but Daviel first devoted himself exclusively to ophthalmology in 1728 (Hirschberg).* The second claim is effectually disposed of by the following extract from a letter addressed in 1752 by Dr Thos. Hope to Dr Clephane, and communicated to the Royal Society(43).

In answer to what is said, that it (the operation of extraction) has been practised before, and that Taylor formerly performed, he (Daviel) endeavours to prove it never was, excepting in cases, where the crystalline had, by some accident, slip(ped) thro' the pupilla into the anterior chamber. . . . In regard to Taylor, he may have attempted, but never did carry it into practice; else he would not have failed to have published it in the numberless publications he has given. I know, that, in 1743, I followed him in Edinburgh for six months, where he performed above 100 operations of the cataract by couching, but never once attempted this way, nor ever mentioned it, but in the case, where the crystalline is lodged in the anterior chamber; which operation has been described by many authors.†

From this quotation it will be seen that, in common with his contemporaries, Taylor practised the removal, by a corneal incision, of lenses which became dislocated into the anterior chamber during the operation of couching. It appears also that his treatment for soft cataracts, which could not be couched, was to break them up and evacuate them by means of a paracentesis. Marteau's(80) description of the method employed when the capsule itself was opaque (i.e. in hypermature cataract?) seems to refer to a procedure of this kind.

* *Graefe-Saemisch Handbuch d. ges. Augenheilk.* XIII, ii, p. 473, 1908.

† This letter should not be cited, as has been done, to prove that Taylor *never* performed extraction. Hope's observations relate to 1743, two years before Daviel's discovery, and five years before his first publication; they only prove that Taylor did not *anticipate* the new operation.

Taylor [he says] first pierces the capsule, passing the point of his blunt needle from behind forward through the pupil, after which he makes an opening in the lower part of the cornea, and inserts a small pair of forceps in order, if necessary, to dilate the aperture in the capsule; he then breaks up and lacerates the capsule, and mixes? [there is an illegible word in the original] it with the aqueous, which is rendered opaque by its particles; or he depresses it along with the crystalline.

Haller(40 a) tells us that Taylor distinguished a form of cataract in which the mass of the crystalline was great; this he considered to be incurable by couching, and recommended its extraction by a corneal incision—probably by the method just described.

Apart from these special cases, however, there is good evidence that for many years Taylor's attitude towards Daviel's operation was hostile. In 1759 he is vaunting a new operation "by which all the Advantages of every Method yet practised, whether by its Extraction or otherwise, are effectually obtained"(9). Still more decisive are his remarks in 1761(19) on a case in which he had couched one lens, the other eye having been already operated on elsewhere by extraction. "The faults of this operation", he says, "cannot appear more evident than in this case, for here there is an unequal cicatrix in the glass of the eye, the pupil is contracted and irregular in its form, and the sight almost useless from the absence of the crystalline, unless by a glass extremely convex; whereas in the eye, where my hand has passed, the glass maintains its healthful transparency, the pupil its natural figure, and the crystalline being preserved in the eye, has useful sight without a glass . . . and with a glass of not near the convexity of that used for the other, he sees with great perfection."

His grandson also tells us that "he sometimes adopted the present mode of extracting the cataract, . . . but abandoned it as less certain and more dangerous than depression"(97).

Stricker(96) states that his objections to extraction in the case of solid cataract were: (1) That it is impossible to foretell the diameter of the lens, and therefore to judge how large the corneal incision should be. (2) That after operation the eye must be closed, which hinders the flow of tears. (3) That the stretching of the pupil to deliver the lens is dangerous. (4, 5) That the large accumulation of aqueous behind the iris, and the concave form which the vitreous must assume are detrimental to vision, whereas if the lens remains in the eye the vitreous takes a convex figure and assumes the function of the displaced crystalline.*

It is not till 1765 that we meet with a definite claim on the part of Taylor to have performed extraction. In an advertisement issued at Rheims(96), he invites the attention of the faculty to the question which is the better operation. For reasons well known to *savans en optique*, vision cannot be so good after extraction as after couching; but the difference can be remedied by glasses. If the cataract is solid he uses both methods with equal success, if fluid in whole or in part, he performs extraction by a method of his own invention. He has had no bad results from couching because he does not wound the nerve (*i.e.* the long ciliary nerve).

This grudging approbation, be it observed, dates from the Chevalier's sixty-third year. The impression produced is certainly that he never performed the operation, but that in later life the pretence of doing so was forced upon him by its increasing vogue and success.

AMAUROSIS

Small blame would attach to Taylor if his views on amaurosis, or "gutta serena", were no more enlightened than those of anyone else before the discovery of the ophthalmoscope. But the

---

* Stricker gives some interesting early statistics of extraction; one surgeon had fourteen failures in thirty-eight cases (nine times atrophy of the globe, five times staphyloma, *i.e.* prolapse?); another had seven instances of staphyloma and four of atrophy in fourteen cases; another had nine total, and three partial, losses in seventeen; Caqué also confesses to very bad results with the new operation. On the other hand, Hope(43) says that Daviel had a hundred successes out of one hundred and fifteen cases, and adds his testimony as an eyewitness, that although the operation lasted two minutes the patient complained of little or no pain, and said he felt no more than a tickling sensation.

book in which he deals with the subject, the *Traité sur les Maladies de l'Organe immédiat de la Vûë*(2) cannot be freed from the imputation of deliberate dishonesty. A parade of knowledge was tolerably safe when his critics must be enveloped in darkness as gross as his own.

Accordingly he divides the diseases of the proper organ of sight into (1) perfect, in which vision is totally lost, the pupil being enlarged or diminished, but immobile, and (2) imperfect, in which vision is not lost, but the movements of the pupil have undergone alteration. Of the perfect he differentiates no fewer than twenty-eight species, founding his descriptions on fantastic groupings of cause, duration, pain, the size of the pupil, the distance of the iris from the cornea, the presence or absence of muscae, etc. In spite of his own definition, he speaks of instances with mobile pupils, and he includes cases associated with glaucoma, and violent inflammation following injury—conditions, as his enemies did not fail to point out, which cannot legitimately be termed "gutta serena". The imperfect are divided into true and false, the true being the above twenty-eight varieties of the perfect before vision is completely lost. In the false imperfect, vision is diminished, but not extinguished, even in the latest stages; the group includes nyctalopia and hemeralopia, and one variety occurs in women after great loss of blood. The actual seat of the disease may be (1) in the brain, which may be too cold, hot, dry, or humid, etc.; or (2) in the chambers of the optic nerve, which "are called the thalami nervorum opticorum", by their "oppression, astriction, affliction, and constipation", etc.; or (3) in the optic nerve or contiguous parts from "compression, decadence, subsidence, expansion, constriction, dryness, or atrophy". An elaborate disquisition is appended on the cause of muscae volitantes; the true variety is due to expansion of the retinal arteries, but oily particles in the aqueous, or opacities in the lens or vitreous may also produce similar appearances.

In later life Taylor seems to have felt that some apology for this book was required, or to have perceived that it had missed its mark with the learned. In 1750 he speaks of it as "a work of my youth, at which time I had not the requisite opportunities for adequate investigation of this subject, which now my daily experience in curing eyes has given me"(4a). By this time he has abandoned the idea that muscae may be due to opacities in the media, because, if the surface of a lens be strewn with fine grains of sand, a clear image is still thrown by it; muscae, therefore, are an affection of the immediate organ of sight.

A subject so obscure offered a tempting field of activity to the charlatan. Already, in 1736, Taylor announces his ability to cure several kinds of gutta serena(3); in later life he rather modifies than expands his pretensions, and in 1761 he limits his claim to "at least one species"(19). According to his own account, his method "consists only in rubbing the lower Part of the Globe with a small Instrument, whose surface is a little unequal, by which the Freedom of the Nerves destined for the Motion of the Pupil is almost instantly recovered . . . and it is on the natural Movements of the Pupil that depends the healthful Protection of Sight"(29). Lecat(45) tells us that the instrument in question took the form of a silver spoon with a rasp fixed to the convexity; we have already seen it in action in the case of Caqué's friend the Canon(80). He sometimes used vigorous massage on the closed eye with the concavity of the same spoon. These procedures were directed specially against the immobility of the pupil. For the amaurosis itself he pricked the muscles with a blunt needle in order that, by their contraction, they might stimulate the inactive nerve(40a, 47). He also bled his patients from the jugular vein, and gave them strong emetics(39).

Before these methods are dismissed as puerilities or worse, it should be stated that there is a considerable body of reputable contemporary testimony not only to their reasonableness, but what is more surprising, to their efficacy, in certain cases. Dr Marteau, of Amiens(80), states that, although previously sceptical, he witnessed a cure in one case, improvement in another, and a failure in a third. While protesting against excessive claims, Mauchart(47) considers that some forms of gutta serena may be curable, and that puncture and friction are not summarily to be rejected, but should rather be imitated, improved, and brought to perfection in a cautious manner; for the nerves of the lid, conjunctiva, and muscles are derived from the third, fourth, fifth and sixth pairs, and these communicate with the nerves in the uvea and around the optic nerve, so that stimulation of one may stimulate the other. He quotes a case of Valsalva's, in which amaurosis was cured by massage of the supra-orbital nerve at its exit; he suggests that on the same principle electricity might be tried in the gutta serena. Lecat(45) also admits the reasonableness of friction. Guérin(39) tells us that Taylor's aim was to obtain prompt, if apparent, cures, by giving a temporary activity to the retina. "He applied a very fine golden file several times to the transparent cornea; the irritation was general, and was communicated to the proper organ of sight, which, under stimulation, became more sensitive for the moment." Taylor then exhibited some object to the patient, who *did*, in fact, see better at the moment, whereupon he *chantoit victoire*, and behaved in the manner described on p. 156. Guérin's considered opinion is that the file does awake the retina to action, and that the prolonged use of active remedies in the form of collyria may, therefore, exercise a similar effect on that membrane, even although it be a little distant.

SQUINT

In his theoretical views on squint Taylor was certainly in advance of his time; indeed, some of his doctrines have an astonishingly modern sound(4 a). He begins by examining and explaining the views of his predecessors—of St Yves, who held that the condition was the result of a too great convexity on one or other side of the centre of the cornea; of Ferrein, who hypothecated an oblique position of the lens; of Porterfield, who combined these two explanations. All these, as well as the view that the most sensitive part of the retina is situated somewhere not on the normal optic axis, lack the confirmation of experience.

Squint, in fact, is nothing but a misdirection of the axis of the eye on looking at objects. If such a misdirection be produced artificially by pressure on the globe, diplopia results, because the image falls on an abnormal area of the retina. Why, then, does this not occur in the subjects of squint? Because many of them see better with one eye than the other, or if they see equally well with both they use one more than the other, and, therefore, direct its axis on to the object. If anything be brought too close to the eyes of a normal person pain is experienced and a squint is induced; but this differs from a true squint in being present only under these conditions. The permanency of a true squint is accounted for by this same unilateral defect; the object is looked at with one eye and the other is directed elsewhere (the meaning seems to be, clearly enough, that the defective eye is free to wander because it is useless for vision). An image is indeed formed in the squinting eye, but it is so weak that it does not hinder the clear vision of the other, just as a strong pressure makes a light pressure imperceptible, or a strong light overcomes a weaker. Moreover, with practice one learns to disregard a second image. Taylor once had the opportunity of observing a man who developed a squint in consequence of an injury to his ocular muscles; at first he was much troubled with diplopia and had to shut one eye in going up and down stairs, but later, although no change in the position of the eye occurred, he gradually learned to overcome his double vision. Again, those who look through a telescope with both eyes open receive an image in the second eye, but neglect it because their attention is directed to the apparently nearer, more distinct image of the other. In reading also a large part of the image is disregarded. The diplopia of drunkenness is due to the irregular action of the muscles.

Taylor knew well also that on covering the sound eye the squinting eye came straight. The observation is said to have been first made by St Yves* in 1722, but apparently it was not generally known, and Taylor's unscrupulous cleverness is shown by the manner in which he exploited it for the deception of the public. When Lecat(45) asked him why he put the bandage on the sound eye "il fit le distrait et ne me repondit rien", not wishing

* Hirschberg ((84), p. 309).

apparently to give away the secret, it was only on thinking the matter over that Lecat remembered having himself observed the phenomenon, and hit upon the satisfactory explanation that the squinting eye was lazy, but had to set to and do its share of the work when the other was occluded.

Taylor's account of the more remote causes, and of the varieties of squint is less original. In children, he says, it is an acquired habit not resulting from a defect of the eye itself or of its muscles, but due to association with squinting persons; or to the bringing of too many objects to their notice at the same time, which causes them to attempt to look simultaneously in different directions; or to their being placed constantly with a window on one side, so that the eyes are kept in a constrained position, and one is preferred before the other; or to a disproportion in the parts of the eye, in which case it cannot be cured; or to a disease elsewhere in the body, in which case also it is frequently incurable. His classification is as follows: (1) One straight eye, the other divergent. (2) Both eyes divergent. (3) One eye straight, the other convergent. (4) One eye directed upwards (9 e).

It would seem, therefore, that Taylor had a very fair knowledge of the influence of defective vision in producing squint, and also of the suppression of the image of the squinting eye. He distinguished clearly between ordinary squint with no defect of movement and paralytic squint due to injury of the ocular muscles. That he had some idea of other forms of paralytic squint is suggested by the following quotation:* "It is, however, not to be denied that all degrees of this infirmity may also be caused by some lesions of the muscles of the globe, such as abnormal configuration, or from some other disease, such as gout . . . by which the equilibrium of the muscles is interfered with" (4 a).

Taylor's title to be regarded as a pioneer in operations upon squint has been so fully examined by Schrön (94), Antonelli (77) and Hirschberg (84), that only a brief reference to the subject need be made in this place.

* Paralytic squint is said to have been recognised by Galen (84).

The facts are these:

(1) From an early period of his career ((66), 1737), he began to advertise that he could cure squint without trouble or danger, and with an invariably good result.

(2) There is contemporary evidence both (a) as to the nature of his proposals and (b) as to the operation which he actually performed.

Eschenbach(38) in 1752 writes: "Some oculists have indeed dreamt that it might be possible to divide in whole or part the rectus muscle of the globe which is chiefly at fault, and by such an operation to cure the squint". This is couched in general terms, but it occurs in a book devoted to the examination of Taylor's pretensions, and follows immediately after an exposition of Taylor's views. The probability that the reference is to Taylor is increased by the following quotation, written two years later (38 a): "Oculists have imagined that squint may be curable by the division of one or other of the muscles of the eye. Taylor did not do so in Rostock". The following passage occurs in a work by Heurmann ((42), 1756): "Taylor has also proposed to cure squint by dividing the belly of the superior oblique muscle; but as squint is not always caused by the contraction of this muscle, and as the inferior oblique, on dividing the superior, pulls the eye over to the opposite side and gives rise to a new kind of squint, and as the recti muscles which often cause squint cannot well be divided on account of their position, it follows that this operation can very seldom be practicable. Few patients also would submit to it, because squint is not so very intolerable, and the operation must be very painful and uncertain in its results".

As to the operation which Taylor actually performed, the best evidence is that of the eyewitness Lecat(45). Taylor, he tells us, took up a fold of the conjunctiva towards the inferior part of the globe by means of a needle threaded with silk, cut it off with scissors, and clapped a plaster on the sound eye; the squinting eye came straight "et chacun criait miracle". When asked the reason for this procedure, he explained that squint was due to a loss of equilibrium of the muscles, and that, in order to re-establish it, the over-powerful muscle must be weakened by dividing one of its nervous filaments of supply. How Lecat thereupon lured Taylor to his undoing has been related on p. 156. The same operation is recognisable in the following passage written by Eschenbach(38 *a*) eleven years later: "The explanation which he gave of his operation, in that he spoke of dividing a nerve, might lead some authors to believe that he wished to deceive the medical public into thinking that he really divided the internal rectus muscle after he had pulled the eye outwards with his conjunctival stitch, but nothing in the facts as communicated justifies such an assumption".

It will be seen that there are here three distinct proposals: to divide (1) the superior oblique, (2) the internal rectus, (3) a nerve supplying the over-powerful muscle. The first of these, if it was ever put forward as a routine treatment for ordinary internal strabismus, was certainly not a very luminous suggestion. It is remarkable, however, that none of these procedures is anywhere mentioned in his books, unless it be in his treatise on strabismus(6), which seems to be lost. In one of his works(9 *c*) squint is placed in the index as a condition which can only be cured by operation. The most probable explanation of this reticence is that he wished to make a mystery of his method, or possibly he thought that it would scarcely bear the light of day. It is true that he freely describes his operation for cataract and the artificial pupil, but these were at best only variations on well-known operations; a surgical cure for squint was something much more novel.

On the whole the impression conveyed is that he recognised clearly that squint was a disturbance of muscle equilibrium; that he conceived the idea that it might be cured by dividing a muscle—and in this conception apparently he is really entitled to the credit of priority; that either with, or very much more probably without, having made the attempt, he became convinced that the operation was impracticable; that in order not to lose his dishonest emoluments he devised the fraudulent procedure described by Lecat; that for the hoodwinking of intelligent onlookers or critics he further invented two stories—first, that he divided a nervous filament; second, that his stitch served to fix the globe while he divided the muscle. However this may be, the proposal to divide a muscle for squint slumbered for nearly a century till it was put into practice on the cadaver by Strohmeyer, on the living in 1838 by Dieffenbach.

IRITIS

The characteristic features of iritis are only dimly perceptible in Taylor's works. He tells us that after a violent inflammation which has been inefficiently treated the connexions of some of the vessels in the framework of the iris near the pupil may be interrupted, in consequence of which the form and position of these vessels is disordered and they become confusedly interlaced. The cicatrix which results may cause occlusion of the pupil ((4 *a*), p. 213). Elsewhere he says that in consequence of a prolonged inflammation the pupil may become small, misshapen, and immovable(9 *e*). He claims to have invented the operation of forming an artificial pupil; but as the operation is Cheselden's and he gives no details, the subject need not be pursued.

SYMPATHETIC OPHTHALMITIS

That Taylor had tolerably sound ideas on the subject of sympathetic ophthalmitis, and also on the impropriety of operating on unilateral cataract, is shown by the following passage(1): "Where there is a Cataract in one Eye, and the other Eye is sound and good, the Patient don't ought to be encourag'd to suffer the diseased Eye to be Couch'd; because the Symptoms which may possibly attend it may be the Occasion of the loss of both". In illustration he reports a case in which mature cataract was present in one eye, incipient in the other. After the first had been couched "The Eye continued clear, and the Patient saw for some Days. At which Time an Inflammation came on, which equally affected both Eyes; and, notwithstanding all I could do to abate it, the Coats and Humors were so thicken'd by it, that the Eye which had the Suffusion [*i.e.* the incipient cataract] in it became totally blind: And some Time after, that which I had couch'd was in like manner entirely depriv'd of Sight; tho' the Cataract remain'd depress'd, and the pupilla perfectly clear".

This was in 1727; in later life, unfortunately, honesty was overcome by greed. In the *Parallel*(29) he tells us that it is an idle opinion, when one eye is lost or in danger, "not to use Means for its Recovery, because such Means may affect the other". Pain, if allowed to continue, is dangerous, but its relief by operation may be the means of saving the second eye; on the other hand, if there is no pain, an operation on one eye cannot affect the other, "more than what's done to the Right Hand can affect the Left". Besides, by his method he avoids "every sensible Part of the least Consequence that has any communication with the opposite Eye".

A case, evidently of sympathetic ophthalmitis with occlusion of the pupil, in which Taylor operated by couching the pupillary membrane, is described by Heister(41). The result was an acute inflammation ending, despite the most vigorous treatment, in atrophy of the globe. Before Taylor is condemned, however, it should be mentioned that Heister himself intended to operate if the patient had not taken matters into his own hands by deserting him for the English oculist(96).

MISCELLANEOUS OPERATIVE MEASURES

Corneal Opacities. In the treatment of corneal opacities Taylor employed two methods. In the first, after inserting a speculum he proceeded to "pare off the Excrescence with a small curv'd knife, leaving as few Inequalities as possible; and having pre-vented an Inflammation by proper Repellents, I blow a powder into the eye, which, assisted by the Motion of the Eyelid, smooths off the Inequalities left by the Knife". The second consisted in scrubbing the eye with a small brush made of barley bristles(1). Duddell(37) adversely criticised the first, but approved and practised the second, which is said to have been introduced by Woolhouse. Lecat(45) informs us that Taylor also used his brush as a means of letting blood in conjunctival affections; he expresses a qualified approval, but doubts whether the results, in the case of corneal cicatrices, are likely to be permanent. A reference to the same treatment is found in the burlesque *Doctor Sartorius Sinegradibus*(70), where, a clergyman having been called in consultation on the doctor's disordered wits, Sartorius "began to brush the Parson's eyes with Bear-awns".*

Ectropion. The dramatic setting of the following description of an ectropion operation deserves to be retained(19):

Being in one of the principal courts abroad, I saw a lady in the drawing-room of a great court, who had the lower lid of her left eye fallen down, by an accident from fire, which left part of her eye uncovered, this defect destroyed the beauty of one of the finest faces I ever saw. I approached her excellency ... and spoke to this effect; "permit me lady to tell you that one half of that face of yours is exquisitely pretty. Well, Sir, she said, and what do you say to the other? Why, the other, Madam, said I, is so much the reverse that it strikes me with horror; how, Sir, said the lady with great quickness; What insolence is this?"

Taylor assured her that he would not have made that severe remark had he not the power of making both sides of her face equally handsome. Having sent for his instruments, therefore, and having retired with the lady to a private apartment, I immediately passed a needle through the skin of the temple, near the lesser angle of the eye, and with my lancet dissected, to about half an inch diameter, the skin of that part from the muscles. Whilst thus employed, her excellency often called out to me, "you hurt me! you hurt me!" And I as often answered, "remember lady, beauty! beauty"! and with this charming word beauty I softened her pain in such a manner that she kept her courage to the end of the operation, which was to draw the edges of the wound together and fix them so by passing the needle threaded through them as to tie them together. Thus I brought that upper [? lower] eyelid into its place without touching it, and after putting

* Bear awns = beards of barley (Jamieson's *Dict. of Scot. Language*).

on the wound now closed, a small plaster, which seemed rather an ornament than a blemish, I conducted the lady back to the courtiers in the palace. Seeing her thus changed, they all appeared astonished, and looked as if this business had been done by some miracle.

Ptosis. His ptosis operation is described as follows: "A married lady of distinction once presented to my care, who had such a defect in her upper eye-lids, that her eyes were almost ever covered, and, when she wanted to see, was obliged to lift her head very high, or to raise her eye-lids by her own hands. By my well-known method of curing this defect, I soon fixed the lady's eye-lids like those of other people, which is by removing a part of these eye-lids, and sewing the lips of the wound delicately together, as in the preceding case".

MISCELLANEOUS OBSERVATIONS

Conical Cornea. In his delineation of conical cornea Taylor seems to have been preceded only by Duddell,* who, in 1736, reported the case of a boy, aged 14 years, who had very prominent corneae, like truncated cones, nystagmus, and a red reflex from the pupil. Taylor not only describes, but figures the condition in an unmistakable manner. "It is", he says, "a change in the form of the cornea by which it takes the form of a cone, whose apex is blunt, but whose base is equal to the diameter of the cornea, which preserves its transparency" ((9), (9e), xc, xci). He calls it Ochlodes, and distinguishes a second form in which the apex is sharp.

Glaucoma. Since glaucoma as now understood did not exist for Taylor, it is superfluous to enter deeply into his speculations on the vaguely differentiated variety of gutta serena which he distinguished under that term. Let the reader make what he can of the following definition:

By a Glaucoma I understand a diseas'd alteration of the Chrystalline, where the Chrystalline maintains one exact equal Continuity thro' all its Parts, with a diseas'd Alteration of its Capsula, attended with

---

* Suppl. to the *Treatise on the Disease of the Horny Coat*, quoted Hirschberg (84), xiv Bd., xxxiii Kap., p. 130.

degrees of a very equal Opacity and Colour, very great Increase of Diameter, preternatural Change of its Consistence, Gravity and Situation; and in its last state with an Elevation, Dilatation, and Immobility of the Pupil, and Gutta Serena.

Later definitions ((9) §§ 160–2, (9 e)) show more clearly that he regarded the condition as being due essentially to a swelling of the lens, but, according to Haller(40 a), he also spoke of a form in which the lens was small and sprang out of its capsule when incised. His account of the cause of the affection is mere jargon; his treatment, "where the Iris and immediate Organ of Sight maintain their healthful Perfection", was couching.

Anophthalmos. This observation occurs among the wonderful tales of the Autobiography(19). In Stockholm he knew a lady who was so affected by seeing her brother's house on fire that she gave birth to a child which seemed as if it had just been burnt, and was born without eyes, "the place where the eyes should be, appearing as consumed with fire".

REPORTS OF INDIVIDUAL CASES

A good idea of Taylor's methods of treatment and point of view on certain subjects may be obtained from his account of the case of Sir Jeremy Sambrooke(22). He published several similar narratives relating the histories of illustrious patients, but no other seems to have survived. The treatise on Sir Jeremy is not, as might perhaps have been expected, a song of triumph, but the defence of a failure. In the dedication he tells us that he is sensibly touched at the disappointment of his hopes, more on Sir Jeremy's account than his own. He has taken great pains with the case, has surmounted most of the difficulties, and has reason to expect an excellent result in the immediate future. He begs him therefore not to dispense with the services "of which you cannot be now deprived, without the greatest Injustice and basest Inhumanity".

Having operated with success upon Sir Jeremy's sister and several others (whose names are given in full), Taylor was called in to the assistance of the Baronet himself. He found the right eye irrecoverably blind from birth; the left lens was opaque, but the pupil was active and there was perception of light. Couching was therefore performed on the left, but to his "extraordinary surprise" there was no restoration of vision. As headaches were also present he concluded that there must be a diseased condition of the brain due to abnormal distension of blood-vessels, and therefore divided the temporal artery, with the result that the headaches ceased and his patient had a confused "Impression of the Object". On the fourth day, however, secondary hæmorrhage ensued, and continued at intervals for twenty days. The dilemma was painful; the hæmorrhage could not be allowed to continue, but if pressure were applied it might bring back the headache and so destroy the sight. Finally, however, the use of a bandage could not be avoided, the bleeding was stopped, but the eye became painful and much inflamed, and a hypopyon formed in spite of repeated general evacuations. At first Taylor was afraid to let out the pus on account of the violence of the inflammation, and also lest it "might have acquired such an Acrimony, as would corrode the Sides of the Aperture in the Cornea". Despite these considerations, however, it became necessary to drain the anterior chamber, which he did by punctures "to the Number of near 20 at different Times", being aware of the danger of iris prolapse if he made a large opening. By these means the hypopyon was got rid of, but in the meantime the "Pupil gradually lost its mobility and Figure, till at last it remained nearly closed"; the iris was also "elevated towards the cornea"; some even asserted—falsely—that the globe "had lost something of its healthful Figure". In the remainder of the work Taylor points out the exceedingly peculiar features of this very straightforward case of operation on a blind eye, infection, occlusion of the pupil, iris bombé, and commencing phthisis bulbi; he proposes the formation of an artificial pupil in the lower part of the iris, and ends with an appeal that he may not be "hindered from the Prosecution of those Measures I have already so successfully (and I think I may venture to say, so rationally) taken".

The vigour of Taylor's treatment, illustrated in the above relation, was condemned in the manifesto of the Royal College of Physicians of Edinburgh(68), where it is stated that the health of many patients had been impaired and their sight made worse by excessive unnecessary evacuations, and other irregular methods of practice. A similar accusation is made by Heister(41). The treatment which evoked these protests in the middle of the eighteenth century must have been drastic indeed. Lecat(45) mentions his use of violent sternutatories, and says he had a collyrium of which a small bottle was sold for a louis.

Such was the Chevalier Taylor. A striking and picturesque figure; of good person and address seemingly, with something not unattractive in his manner; at any rate wholly unembarrassed by any diffidence in his dealings with the great. An unparalleled liar, pre-eminent among charlatans in the arts of advertisement; with a natural aptitude for the grand style; rapacious in acquiring, profuse, but not generous in expending. His literary gifts were not despicable; he seems to have possessed a sense of humour, and he could give and take in an encounter of wits; his public oratory must surely have been something less lugubrious than the account of his appearance at Northampton (p. 148) would indicate. His showy qualities undoubtedly imposed upon many intelligent contemporaries, but by the more discerning he seems to have been regarded as an amusing rascal. In professional matters his knowledge was good; he was a shrewd observer and not without original ideas; but his actual practice was deeply tainted with the dishonest arts of the quack. Many elements go to the formation of the complete charlatan—bombast, effrontery, dishonesty, ignorance. All these qualities Taylor showed in perfection—except ignorance, and this is his chief condemnation.

BIBLIOGRAPHY AND REFERENCES

It is impossible to reconstruct a fully authentic bibliography of Taylor's works. His own list, published in the *Travels and Adventures* (19), numbers forty-five, with the promise of several more, but, as might be expected, it is inflated to the utmost extent by the inclusion of the same work in various guises and in different languages— perhaps also by the manufacture for the occasion of fictitious titles. Moreover he sometimes gives, not the real title, but only a descriptive sentence in English, which sometimes renders difficult the identification of books published abroad. Even in the case of works which are still extant there are a good many inaccuracies as to date of publication, etc. The following bibliography is founded, *faute de mieux*, on the list in the *Travels and Adventures*, supplemented and corrected so far as possible from the works themselves, and from a similar list in the *Racolta dell' opere scritte* (30). In the case of extant works the real title-page has been substituted for Taylor's description.

TREATISES AND MONOGRAPHS

(1) An Account | of the | Mechanism | of the | Eye. Wherein its Power of Refracting the Rays | of Light, and Causing them to Converge at the | Retina, is consider'd: With an Endeavour to | ascertain the true Place of a Cataract, and | to shew the good or ill Consequences of a Judicious | or Injudicious Removal of it. | By John Taylor, Surgeon in Norwich. |

> Hear him ye Deaf, and all ye Blind behold!
> He from thick Films shall purge the Visual Ray,
> And on the sightless Eye-Ball pour the Day.

Norwich: | Printed by Henry Cross-grove, and Sold by the Book- | sellers of London and Norwich, 1727.

(Copies in libraries of R.L.O.H., B.M., R.C.S., R.S.M., F.F.P.S.G.*)

Dedicated to Mr William Cheselden. For remarks see number (4) below.

(2) Traité | sur | les Maladies | de | l'Organe immédiat | de la Vûë. | Adressé à Messieurs de l'Académie Royale | des Sciences à Paris. | Par Jean Taylor, Docteur en Médecine, | Chirurgien & Oculiste, & membre de la Faculté | de Médecine de l'Université de Basle en Suisse. | Qui dat videre, dat vivere. Cic. | A Paris, | Chez Prault fils, Quay de Conti, à la | Charité. | MDCCXXXV. | Avec Approbation & Privilege du Roy. |

(Copies in B.M., T.C.D., F.F.P.S.G.)

An advertisement states that this is only a small instalment of a complete treatise. The contents of the work are sufficiently analysed at p. 180.

(2 *a*) An English edition of this work is said to have been published in 1743. I have been unable to find a copy.

(3) A new | Treatise | on the | Diseases | of the | Chrystalline Humour | of a | Human Eye: | Or, of the | Cataract and Glaucoma. | With a | New Theory of their Causes, and an En | deavour to demonstrate that there are no membranous | Cataracts; but that all Cataracts are from an Altera | tion of the chrystalline Humour itself. | With | An exact Description of a new

* R.L.O.H. = Royal London Ophthalmic Hospital. B.M. = British Museum. R.C.S. = Royal College of Surgeons, England. R.S.M. = Royal Society of Medicine. T.C.D. = Trinity College, Dublin. F.F.P.S.G. = Faculty of Physicians and Surgeons, Glasgow.

and more success | ful Method of making the operations necessary to the | Removal of the several Species of these Diseases. | Humbly address'd to her Majesty. | To which is prefix'd, | a letter to the Physicians and | Surgeons of London and Westminster. | Qui dat videre, dat vivere. Cic. | By John Taylor, M.D. Oculist, | Fellow of the College of Physicians of | Basle in Switzerland, of the Imperial Academy | of Cologn in Germany, and of the Society of | Liege and Rheims. | London: | Printed for James Roberts, near the Oxford-Arms | in Warwick-Lane. M DCC XXXVI.

(Copies in R.L.O.H., B.M., T.C.D., R.C.S., F.F.P.S.G.)

The contents are sufficiently indicated in the section of the present paper on cataract, p. 173.

(4) Le Mechanisme | ou | le Nouveau Traité | de l'Anatomie du Globe de l'Oeil, | avec l'usage de ses differentes | parties, & de celles qui lui sont | contiguës. | Orné de Planches gravées en Taille-douce. | Dédié à Monsieur le Premier Medecin | du Roy, | Par Jean Taylor, M.D. | Oculiste du Roy de la Grande Bretagne. | Qui dat videre, dat vivere. | A Paris | Chez Michel-Estienne David, Libraire Quay des Augustins, à la | Providence. | MDCCXXXVIII. | Avec Approbation & Privilege du Roy.

(Copies in B.M., T.C.D., F.F.P.S.G.)

(4 a) Johann Taylors | Ritters, Doctors der Arzneykunst, | Seiner Grossbritannischen Majestät, und verschiedener | andern Durchlauchtigsten Fürsten hochbestallten Augenarztes; | wie auch Mitgliedes vieerEuropäischen berühmten Academien der Wissenschaften, &c., &c. | MECHANISMUS | oder | Neue Abhandlung | von der künstlichen Zusammensezung | des Menschlichen | Auges | und den besondern Nuzen desselben, sowohl | vor sich, als in Absicht der anliegenden Theile, | nebst | seiner Art, dessen Krankheiten | zu heilen, | Wie Er solche bey einer mehr als zwanzigjährigen | Erfahrung seiner durch Europa glüklich gethanen | Augencuren bewährt befunden. | Mit den dazu gehörigen Kupfertafeln. | Unter Königlich-Pohlnisch- und Chur-Sächsischer | allergnädigsten Freyheit, und ausdrüklichen Bewilligung | des Verfassers ins Deutsche übersetz. | Qui dat videre, dat vivere. | Frankfurt am Mayn, | bey Stoks seel. Erben und Schilling. 1750.

(Copies in R.L.O.H., R.S.M., F.F.P.S.G.)

These works are dedicated to Dr Chicoyneau, first physician to the King of France. The German edition has also a dedication to the "Konigliche Gesellschaft den Naturforscher zu Edenburg".

(4 b) A Spanish edition of the same work is said to have been published at Madrid in 1738, and

(4 c) An English edition is promised in 1743 (advertisement in *Jeremy Sambrooke*, No. 22). Whether it ever appeared I do not know.

(4 d) A Danish edition at Copenhagen in 1752 (1753, according to the *Racolta* (30)).

(4 e) An Italian edition of the same work is possibly indicated by the following entry in the *Travels and Adventures*:

"A Treatise on the Eye & its defects; with many figures. Italian. 8vo. Trent. 1755".

The German edition of this book is merely a translation from the French, but the English *Mechanism of the Eye* (1) is an entirely different work. Excluding the preface, the latter contains forty-seven pages, and gives only a brief account of the anatomy and dioptrics of the eye, a discussion of the true seat of cataract, and a description of an ordinary couching operation with its possible complications. It is free from extravagant claims, admits indebtedness to Cheselden and a certain "ingenious gentleman", and propounds sane views on the advisability of operating on unilateral cataract and on the dangers of sympathetic ophthalmitis.

The French *Mechanisme*, on the other hand, is a much more elaborate work, and more nearly approximates to a complete textbook than any other of the Chevalier's writings. Taylor himself considered this and the 243 *Diseases* (9) his best works. It comprises the substance of the *Mechanisme*, the *Traité sur les Maladies de l'Organe immédiat de la Vûë*, and the *Treatise on Cataract and Glaucoma*, and anticipates, in the form of a "hundred questions", the main points of the *Impartial Inquiry* (7). The anatomical portion is much fuller, and contains sections on the eyelids and lacrymal passages, and on the vessels and nerves of the globe; the physiological is mostly new, and deals with such subjects as the origin of the aqueous, the nourishment of the lens and vitreous, the movements of the pupil, binocular vision, etc. The sections on optics and refraction are greatly enlarged, and illustrated with excellent figures—one of the earliest examples, according to Hirschberg (84), of the inclusion of these subjects in an ophthalmic textbook. The operation is now the elaborate procedure first described in the *Treatise on Cataract and Glaucoma*. The author's views on strabismus have been analysed at p. 182. The work concludes with a systematic description, under 263 headings, of all the diseases of the globe and its adnexa. In a general way this follows the same lines as the 243 *Diseases*, which were afterwards the subject of a separate book and atlas (see Nos. (9) and (9 e)), but without the fantastic nomenclature of the later publications. A bibliography of fifty-two authorities on the anatomy, and of eighty-five on the diseases, of the eye is appended.

The German edition of 1750 contains also the 243 *Diseases* under the title, *Kurze Anleitung zu den Vorlesungen*, etc. (see No. (9 c)), and also a translation of the *Syllabus Cursus Anatomiae*, etc., here entitled *Kurzer Begrif einer Anatomischer Abhandlung*, etc. (see Nos. (34), (34 b)).

(5) An Essay on the Action of the Muscles of the Globe of the Eye. In Portuguese. 8vo. Lisbon. 1739 (1738, according to the *Racolta* (30)).

Mentioned in *Travels and Adventures*. No copy known to be extant.

(6) A Treatise on that Defect known by the name of Strabismus, or Squinting. Portuguese. 8vo. Lisbon. 1740 (1739, according to the *Racolta* (30)).

Mentioned in *Travels and Adventures*. No copy known.

(7) An Impartial Inquiry into the Seat of the Immediate Organ of Sight: *viz.* Whether the Retina or Choroides. Being the Subject of a Lecture, in a Course lately given on the Nature and Cure of the Diseases of the Eye. To which is annexed, Five and Forty Queries on this controverted subject. Submitted to the Examination of the Curious.

The title-page is missing from the copy in the British Museum, but the above is taken from an advertisement in *The Case of Sir Jeremy Sambrooke*. The work is dedicated to Dr Burton, from Great Queen Street, Lincoln's Inn Fields. May 17th, 1743.

(7a) An "Essay on Vision", mentioned in the *Travels and Adventures* as being published in Berlin in 1750, may be the same work.

(7b) An Italian edition seems to be indicated by the following entry, "An Essay on the Seat of Vision, with Reflections on the Consequences of determining that Important Question. 8vo. Bologna. 1753".

Contents analysed at p. 168.

(Copy in B.M.)

(8) A Treatise on the Make and Beauty of the Eye, etc. In English. 8vo. London. 1743.

Mentioned in *Travels and Adventures*. No copy known.

(9) An exact Account | of | Two Hundred and forty-three Diseases, | to which the Eye and its Coverings are exposed. | All copied after Nature. | In the Order many Years given, in various Languages, *viz.* | Latin, French, Italian, Portuguese, &c., &c. In the | several Courts, and in Presence of Crowned Heads, | Sovereign Princes, and in many of the most celebrated | Academies, Universities, and Societies of the Learned. | Being the Produce of the greatest Experience, long and most ex | tensive Practice, (in the Cure of distempered Eyes,) of any in the Age we live. The Author the Chevalier | John Taylor, Ophthalmiater, Pontifical, Impe | rial, and Royal *viz.* | To his present Majesty,—To the Pontifical and Imperial Courts, | —To the Kings of Poland, Denmark, and Sweden, &c.—To the | several Electors of the Holy Empire,—To the Royal Infant Duke | of Parma,—To the Prince Royal of Poland,—To the Prince Royal | Charles of Lorrain,—To the Princes of Saxe-Gotha, Orange, | Brunswick, Anspach, Bareith, Hesse Cassel, Mecklenburg, | Modena, Bavaria, Holstein, Liege, Zerbst, Salts- burg, | Georgia, &c., and to almost all other crowned Heads and Sovereign | Princes of Europe,—Professor in Optics,—Member of the most cele | brated Academies, Universities, and Societies of the Learned, *viz.* In | France, Spain, Portugal, Russia, Italy, Germany, Poland; and, in gene | ral, in all the Holy Empire, in Sweden, Denmark, Switzerland, Holland, | Netherlands, &c.—Raised to the Dignity of Citizen and Noble of | Rome, by a public Act, in the name, and with the Voice of the Se | nate and People,—Fellow of that College of Physicians, and of the | Colleges of Padua, Pavia, Ratisbon, Gottingen, &c.—Doctor of Phy | sic and Doctor of Chirurgery in many of the most eminent Universi | ties—Chevalier in several of the first Courts of the World,—and Au | thor of forty-four

Works on the Art of restoring and preserving Sight; | all written by himself in several languages.—Who has been not only | several Times in every Town in these Kingdoms, (*viz.* Great Britain | and Ireland) but in every Kingdom, Province, State, and City, of the | least consideration,—in every Court, and presented to every crown | ed Head and Sovereign Prince in all Europe, without Exception. | Qui Visum, Vitam dat. | Edinburgh. | Printed by Robert Fleming. M.DCC.LIX. |

Dedicated to the President and Fellows of the Royal College of Physicians at Edinburgh.

(Copies in R.C.S., R.S.M., T.C.D., F.F.P.S.G.)

The above title-page is taken from the English edition published at Edinburgh in 1759. The work also appears in the following forms:

(9 *a*) A Latin edition. London. 1743.

(9 *b*) A somewhat enlarged English edition. Edinburgh. 1744.

(9 *c*) Incorporated with the German *Mechanismus des Auges*, 1750 (4 *a*), under the following title:

Kurze Anleitung | zu den | Vorlesungen | über die Krankheiten | des | Augapfels | und dessen nahe liegenden | Theilen.

(9 *d*) An Italian edition thus mentioned in the *Travels and Adventures*: An exact description of all the Defects of Sight, all in the order of the most regular Science; addressed to the learned Dr Morgagni, Professor in Padua. 8vo. Venice. 1755 (1757, according to the *Racolta* (30)).

(9 *e*) As an Atlas in Latin and German, with the following title: Johannis Taylor, Equ. | Med. Doct. | Imp. Reg. et Princ. plur. Ophthalmiatri, | plurimarumque Academiarum Socii, | NOVA | NOSOGRAPHIA | OPHTHALMICA; | hoc est | accurata Recensio | Ducentorum et quadraginta trium affectuum, | qui | Oculum humanum | partesque vicinas | ullo modo laedere aut ipsum visum adimere | possunt; | Iconibus | artificiosissime sculptis | et | Coloribus ad vivum expressis incredibili accuratione | illustrata. | Hamburgi et Lipsiae, Impensis hæredum Grund & Holle, | MDCCLXVI.

(Copies in R.S.M., F.F.P.S.G.)

(9 *f*) A French edition of the 243 *Diseases* is mentioned by Stricker. Published at Angers, 1766.

In this work the diseases of the eyelids, lacrymal passages, conjunctiva and cornea are usually fairly recognisable; those of the iris much less so; while those which are attributed to enlargement and diminution of the lens and to disease of the immediate organ of sight are mostly fantastic. But however fanciful the description an elaborate Greek name is not lacking, the nomenclature showing, according to Stricker (96), little knowledge of that language, and being disfigured by many misprints.

The *Nosographia* is a sumptuous work in folio, in which illustrations of the 243 *Diseases* are set out on 22 plates surrounded by florid borders. In a preliminary plate a winged female figure points to a blank shield, while underneath, sitting on a cloud, a Cupid prepares to operate on a huge eye with a couching needle; above, two Cupids exhibit a page of the work, while a third flies in the air flourishing a knife. The figures themselves are fairly well executed, but it must be confessed that those which profess to illustrate such conditions as "lack of tears", nystagmus (termed "Hippos"), nyctalopia, hemeralopia, etc., are more pleasing than instructive. The phrase in the title-page "coloribus ad vivum expressis" does not apply to the copies examined by Hirschberg or myself, but apparently Stricker had seen an example in which "unnaturally harsh" colour had been used. In spite of its defects, however, the book is apparently entitled to the credit of being the first attempt at an Atlas of Ophthalmology. It contains an accurate figure and description of conical cornea (see p. 190).

(10) A Treatise on the Anatomy of the Eye and its Coverings, with Figures; a picture of the author, engraved by the best hand. German. 8vo. Dresden. 1750.

Mentioned in *Travels and Adventures*. No copy known, unless this be another name for the *Kurzer Begrif einer Anatomischen Abhandlung* (34b), which, however, contains no figures, and was published at Frankfurt and Leipzig.

(11) A Dissertation on the Eye, etc. Frankfurt. 1751.

This might be supposed to be the *Mechanismus des Auges*, the date of which is erroneously given as 1751 in Taylor's list; but it is there mentioned as a separate work.

(12) A Treatise on a new Method of recovering Sight, lost by a Vice of the crystalline Humour of the eye; addressed to His Eminence the Prince Cardinal Alexander Albani. Italian. 8vo. Pessaro. 1756.

(12a) The following would appear to be the same work in a different dress:

A Work, intitled, a new Method of restoring Sight when lost, by a Vice in the crystalline Humour of the Eye; an Operation entirely new, of the Invention of the Chevalier Taylor, and by him only practised. This Method occasions little or no Pain, requires no Alteration of Diet, and admits not even the Possibility of a Relapse; all of which have been proved by an extraordinary Number of Instances; on these Occasions the Faculty and the Learned, are always invited, in all places where the Author passes. Italian. 4to. Milan. 1756.

Mentioned in *Travels and Adventures*. No copies known.

(13) A Dissertation on the Art of preserving healthful Sight; addressed to his Serene Highness the Duke of Modena. Italian. 8vo. Milan. 1756.

(13a) An English translation of this work is promised in the *Travels and Adventures*. Whether it ever appeared I do not know.

Mentioned in *Travels and Adventures*. No copy known.

(14) A Treatise on the Nature of those Defects, known by the Name of Weakness of Sight, and the manner of Cure; with a critical Enquiry on all

that has been said by the Antients as well as Moderns on that important Subject. Italian. 8vo. Venice. 1756.

Mentioned in *Travels and Adventures*, where also an English translation is promised. No copies known.

(15) A Dissertation on the Art of restoring the healthful Position of the Eye, lost by a Vice known by the Name of Strabismus, with many figures; addressed to the Royal Infant Duke of Parma. Italian. 4to. Milan. 1756.

Mentioned in *Travels and Adventures*. No copy known.

(16) Considerations on certain Defects of the Eye; where the Sight is entirely lost, and no more to be pretended with judgment, than to remove the deformity. Italian. 4to. Venice. 1756 (1757, according to the *Racolta* (30)).

Mentioned in *Travels and Adventures*. No copy known.

(17) Morbi Oculorum in Systema compendiosum redacti. D. D. Joannis Taylor. Eq. sum. pont. imp. reg. & princ. plur. ophthal. plurimarumque Acad. Soc. &c. 4to. Rome. 1757.

(17a) In the *Travels and Adventures* an English version of what is probably the same work is referred to as being "ready for the Press". An universal Treatise on the Nature and Cure of the Disease in the Eye, containing not only the Practice of all of any Eminency in every Nation in Europe, who have more particularly applied to this most excellent Branch of Physic, but that of the Author's, with all his new Discoveries, whether by Operation or otherwise, most faithfully related; the produce by much of the greatest Experience in the Cure of distempered Eyes, of any in the Age we live. Folio.

No copies known.

AUTOBIOGRAPHICAL

(18) Détails des Motifs pour lesquels le Chevalier Jean Taylor, Docteur en Médecine, Professeur en Optique, Membre, Associé et Agregé de plusieurs Universités, Facultés et Sociétés de Savans en Europe, Médecin Oculiste de S. M. le Roy de la Grande Bretagne, de LL. AA. SS^mes et Royale le Prince et Princesse d'Orange, de S. A. R. Monseigneur le Duc Charles de Lorraine, de LL. AA. S^mes Mgr le Prince Guillaume de Hesse et le Duc Fréderic de Saxe-Gotha, ne s'est pas arreté dans les pais de Brandenbourg. 8vo. Berlin, printed by Etienne de Bourdeaux. 1750.

This work, which I have been unable to consult, contains an account of the Chevalier's adventures with Frederick the Great, as related on p. 142. It is mentioned by Stricker (96).

(19) The History of the | Travels and Adventures | of the Chevalier John Taylor, Ophthalmiater; | Pontifical—Imperial and Royal—The Kings | of Poland, Denmark, Sweden, the Electors of the holy | Empire—the Princes of Saxegotha, Mecklenburg, Anspach, Brunswick, Parma, Modena, Zerbst, Lo | raine, Saxony, Hesse Cassel, Holstein, Salzbourg, Ba | viere, Liege, Bareith, Georgia, etc. Pr. in Opt. C. of Rom. M.D.—C. D.—

Author of 45 works in dif | ferent languages: the Produce of upwards of thirty | years, of the greatest practice in the Cure of distempered Eyes, of any in the age we live—Who has been in every Court, Kingdom, Province, State, | City and Town of the least Consideration in all Europe, without exception. | Written by himself. | This work contains all most worthy of the Attention | of a Traveller—also a Dissertation on the Art of pleasing, | with the most interesting Observations on the Force of Prejudice; number-less Adventures as well among Nuns | and Friars, as with Persons of high Life; with a De | scription of a great Variety of the most admirable Rela | tions which, though told *in his well known peculiar Manner,* each one is strictly true and within the Che | valier's own Observations and Know-ledge.—Interspersed | with the Sentiments of the crown'd Heads, etc. in Favour of | his Enterprizes; and an Address to the Public showing | that his Profession is distinct and independent of every other Part of Physic. | Introduced by an humble Appeal, of the Author, to the Sovereigns of Europe. | Addressed to his only Son. | Vol. 1. | Qui Visum Vitam dat. | London. | Printed for J. Williams, on Ludgate Hill. 1761.

(Copies in B.M., R.C.S.)

The work is nominally in three volumes, but the second and third are paginated continuously, and were published together in 1762. The second is dedicated to David Garrick, the third to the Merchants of London. The book is a farrago of bombast, lies, impertinences and frivolous anecdotes, yet, in Johnson's phrase, "sprightly", and not lacking in strokes of shrewd observation. The copy in the library of the Royal College of Surgeons probably belonged to the Chevalier himself. It is elaborately bound, and on the fly-leaf there is a magnificent coat-of-arms in blue and gold, repre-senting a shield decorated with shells and ermine; above a lion rampant on a helmet holds a shell (? the pilgrim's cockle-shell, in reference to the Author's wandering life). The whole is surrounded by his favourite motto, "Qui Visum Vitam dat", and the book bears the signature J. S. Taylor, probably the Chevalier's great-grandson, John Stirling Taylor.

(20) Anecdotes de la Vie du Chevalier de Taylor, extraites de ses Voyages publiés depuis peu, dediées à la très-haute et très-puissante Princesse Son Altesse, Sérénissime Madame la Princesse de Georgia, Tante du Sérénissime Prince Héraclés de Georgia. Imprimé pour l'Auteur. 4to. 16 pp.

This abbreviated version of the *Travels and Adventures* is mentioned by Stricker (96). I have been unable to find a copy.

To these should perhaps be added his little piece in Italian on "The Art of Making Love with Success" (see p. 140).

REPORTS OF INDIVIDUAL CASES

(21) A Treatise on the extraordinary Disorder and Recovery of Sight, of Don A. de Saldana, Vice-Roy of the Indies. Portuguese. 8vo. Lisbon. 1739.

Mentioned in *Travels and Adventures.* No copy known.

(22) The | Case | of | Sir Jeremy Sambrooke, | Baronet, | Fairly and Impartially Stated. | Containing | a full and exact Account of the Singular | Disorder in the Eye of this Gentle | man. With | a faithful Relation of the great Variety of un | common Circumstances attending his | Cure. | And | a clear Demonstration of the highest Probability of | his perfect Recovery. | Humbly Inscrib'd to Himself. | By J. Taylor, Doctor of Physick; Oculist to his | Majesty; and Member of several of the Colleges of Phy | sicians in Foreign Parts. | Qui dat Videre, dat Vivere. | London: | Printed for J. Crockatt, near Garraway's Coffee House in | Exchange-Alley; and sold by M. Cooper, at the Globe, | in Pater-noster-Row. 1743. | (Price Six-pence.)

(Copies in R.L.O.H., B.M.)
Contents analysed at p. 191.

(23) An exact Description of the singular Disorder, and of the Recovery of Sight, of the Countess of Windischgratz. German. Berlin. 1750.
Travels and Adventures. No copy known.

(24) A Dissertation on the singular Disorder and Recovery of Sight of his Serene Highness the Duke of Mecklenburg, by the Chevalier Taylor. German. 8vo. Hamburg. 1752.
Travels and Adventures. No copy known.

(25) An exact Description of the singular Disorder and Recovery of Sight of the illustrious Lady Nariskin, of the Imperial Family of Russia. Russian. 8vo. Moscow. 1754 (1753 according to the *Racolta* (30)).
Travels and Adventures. No copy known.

(26) Considerations on the extraordinary Disease and Recovery of Sight of the Princess of Georgia, serenissime, Aunt to the Prince Heraclius, supposed to be the present Sophy of Persia. Russian. 8vo. Moscow. 1754 (1753 according to the *Racolta* (30)).
Travels and Adventures. No copy known.

(27) An exact Description of the singular Disorder and Recovery of Sight of her Highness the Princess Justiniana, by the Chevalier Taylor. Italian. 8vo. Rome. 1756.
Travels and Adventures. No copy known.

(28) A Description of the singular Disorder, and of the Recovery of Sight of the celebrated Father Cremona, General of the Order, called the School of Piety, by means of an Artificial Pupil, of the Invention of the Chevalier Taylor; and this in the presence of the late Pope Benedict the XIVth. Italian. 4to. Rome. 1756.
Travels and Adventures. No copy known.

ADVERTISEMENTS, TESTIMONIALS, SUMMARIES OF
LECTURES, PROPOSALS FOR TREATISES, ETC.

(29) A | Parallel, | between | The late Celebrated Mr Pope, | and | Dr Taylor, | Oculist | to the King of Great Britain. | With | various Observations on the Proceedings of Dr Taylor | for near Twenty Years, not only in his Tour through these Kingdoms, but | most parts of Europe. | Address'd | to the Gentlemen, the Ladies, the Clergy, and all of Literature | and Distinction who would be acquainted with his Lectures, Ope | rations, and Success. Wherein | The Reasons of all,—with the many Advantages of a publick Concern from | his Undertakings, are accurately and impartially consider'd. | By a Physician. | Invidia Siculi non invenere Tyranni | Majus Tormentum. Hor. | Printed for the Author. 1748.
    (Copies in B.M., R.S.M.)

(30) Racolta | dell' opere | scritte, e pubblicate | in differenti Lingue, | ed in varie Parti dell' Europa ec. ec. | dal Cavaliere Giovanni di Taylor | (A slip pasted on has a good portrait of the Chevalier with the following inscription and Latin verses) Io: Taylor Eq: sum: pont: imp: reg: et Pr: pl: ophthal: plurimarumque acad. Soc. mult. oper: auct: &c:

> O tu qui terris ades Esculapius alter
> Carus et Europae Regibus et populis:
> Cujus et innumeris Lucem mortalibus almam
> Restituit toties prodigiosa manus:
> Invidiam sanare nequis pulcherrima luscis
> Aspicit ac torvis quae tua Facta oculis.

Verzeichniss | Deren | geschriebenen, und schon kundgemachten Werken | In unterschiedlichen Sprachen, und Theilen der Welt &c. &c. | von dem | Cavalier Joan von Taylor.
    The date is given conjecturally in the British Museum Catalogue as 1758. For analysis of contents see p. 146.

(31) Testimonia, Seu Attestationes, Quibus Cathedratici, caeterique Doctores facultatis Medicinae Professi, Regiae, insignisque Universitatis Conimbricae Lusitaniae, de Operationibus, methodoque oculorum infirmitatibus medendi Joannis Taylor, Medicinae Doctoris, Britannicaeque Maiestatis Physici Ocularii, Attestantur, suasque sententias exponunt, Excelso D. D. Joanni V. Lusitaniae Regi Humillime oblata.
    Advertised in *The Case of Sir Jeremy Sambrooke* as being "now in the Press".

(32) The judgment of crowned Heads, Sovereign Princes and Universities of Europe, on the Enterprizes of Chevalier Taylor. German. 8vo. Augusta. 1755 (1754, according to the *Racolta* (30)).

(33) The Sentiments of the late most high Pontiff Benedict the XIVth, her Imperial Majesty, and of almost all the crowned Heads and Sovereign

Princes in Europe, on the Happy Enterprizes of Chevalier Taylor. Italian. 4to. Milan. 1758.

These Sentiments and Judgments seem to have been published in pamphlet form for distribution as advertisements. They are also given as footnotes in the *Travels and Adventures*.

(34) Syllabus | Cursus Anatomiae, | Infirmitatum | atque | Operationum | Globi ocularis, | et partium contiguarum. | D. D. Josepho Cervy, | Regiae majestatis catholicae | Praeclarissimo Medico Primario, | Meritissimoque Praesidi, Protomedicatûs | Regnorum Hispaniae, etc. | Dicatus à | D. D. Joanne Taylor, M.D. | Regisque magnae Britanniae | Medico Oculario, | Multisque in Academicis celeberrimis Socio | Authore. | Qui dat videre, dat vivere. | Londini: Impensis T. Cooper, ad insigne Globi, in Vico | dicto Pater Noster Row, | MDCCXLIII. | (Pretium 1s. 6d.)
   (Copy in R.C.S.)

(34a) An English edition. Mentioned in (34b).

(34b) A German edition, incorporated with the *Mechanismus des Auges* (4a), with the following title:
   Kurzer Begrif | einer | Anatomischen Abhandlung, | von den | Gebrechen und Heilungs | arten des menschlichen | Auges, | und dessen nahe liegenden Theilen, | beschreiben von | Johann Taylor, | Ritters, Doct. der Arzney-Kunst | Sr. Königl. Gross-Britanischen Maj. | und viel andern Durchlauchtigsten Fürsten, | hochbestalter Augen-Arzt, wie auch Mit-Glied | vieler berühmten Europäischen Academien | der Wissenschaften &c. &c. | Mit dessen | Ausdrüklicher Genehmhaltung, | nach der Lateinisch- und Englischen | Ausgabe ins deutsche übersetzt. | Qui dat videre, dat vivere. | Frankfurt und Leipzig, | bey Stoks Erben und Schilling. | 1750.

(34c) A Swedish edition, described as follows in the *Travels and Adventures*:
   A Syllabus etc. for the Author's publick Academies, in the Order given in various Courts and Universities abroad. Swedish. 8vo. Stockholm. 1753.

(34d) An Italian edition, mentioned in *Travels and Adventures*.

Considerations on a Course of Lectures, and the means of preserving healthful Sight; many years given in a stile, as well for the learned in general, as for those who have knowledge of the Science of the Author. Italian. 4to. Naples. 1756.

The pith of this work lies in a prefatory address to the reader, consisting of sententious maxims in praise of diligence, and in reprehension of sloth, which is the death of the soul. Rejecting the false lights of his predecessors, the author has laboured till he has found an infallible method, applicable easily, without danger, at all times, and to all diseases of the crystalline. Interlarded with the text are numerous Latin tags, which, for the benefit of the vulgar, he condescends to translate, in the German edition, into vernacular verse. In the few remaining pages the headings of the sections and paragraphs of the proposed treatise are set forth.

(35) Considerations on a Treatise universal on the Eye and its Defects, etc. Italian. 8vo. Trent. 1755 (1754 according to the *Racolta*).

This universal treatise appears to have been still *in nubibus* in 1762, when it is said to be "ready for the Press" under the following title:

An Universal Treatise on the Nature and Cure of the disease in the Eye, containing not only the Practice of all of any Eminency in every Nation in Europe, who have more particularly applied to this most excellent Branch of Physic, but that of the Author's, with all his new Discoveries, whether by Operation or otherwise, most faithfully related: the Produce by much of the greatest experience in the Cure of distempered Eyes, of any in the Age we live. English. Folio.

A Latin edition is promised, after which the work will be published in all European languages. Probably it never appeared. The only known work of date subsequent to 1762 seems to be the *Nosographia* (1766).

Examples of the Chevalier's handbill advertisements may be consulted under the following references: *Ann. d'Oc.* (76), Antonelli (77), Dureau (80), v. Duyse (81), Hirschberg (84), Nichols (85).

CONTEMPORARY REFERENCES

(Arranged alphabetically, and, for convenience of reference, numbered continuously with the "Works")

ESTIMATES OF CONTEMPORARIES

I. *Medical.*

(36) CAQUÉ. See under Dureau (80).

(37) DUDDELL, B. Treat. of Horny Coat of Eye. Preface, p. iv and p. 204. 1729.

(37a) *Idem.* An Appendix to the Treat. of Horny Coat. Pp. 9 and 52. 1735. (Quoted by Hirschberg (84).)

(38) ESCHENBACH, D. C. E. Gegründeter Bericht von dem Erfolg der Operationen d. englischen Okulisten, Ritter Taylors, in verschiedenen Städten Teutschlands, besonders in Rostock. 1752. (Quoted by Schrön (94) and Hirschberg (84).)

(38a) *Idem.* Chirurgie. Leipzig. 1754.

(39) GUÉRIN. Traité sur les Maladies des Yeux. Lyons and Paris. Pp. 262 and 276. 1770.

The German edition of this work is entitled Versuch über die Augenkrankheiten. Frankfurt and Leipzig. Pp. 242 and 255. 1773.

(40) HALLER, A. VON. Commercium liter. univ. Pp. 73 and 353. 1734 or ? 1735. (Quoted by Stricker (96) and Hirschberg (84).)

(40a) *Idem.* Bibliotheca Chirurgica II. Pp. 80 and 172. 1775.

(41) HEISTER, E. F. Besondere Nachricht wegen des im Frühjahr Anno 1735 in Holland so sehr gerühmten englischen Oculisten D. Taylors und seiner von ihm verrichteten sehr merkwürdigen, aber höchst unglücklichen Augen-curen nebst andern Nachrichten von diesem Oculisten. Helmstädt. Bey Christ. Fr. Weygand. 1736. (Quoted by Stricker (96).)

(42) HEURMANN, D. GEORG. Abhandl. d. vornehmsten chirurgischen Operationen am menschlichen Koerper, etc. 2 vols. Copenhagen and Leipzig. 1754 (2nd vol. 1756). Vol. II, p. 538. (Quoted by Schrön (94) and Antonelli (77).)

(43) HOPE, THOS. Phil. Trans. vol. XLVII, p. 532, 1751–2.

(44) J. S. Dr Taylor couched for a Cataract. Wherein the Absurdity of his New Treatise on the Diseases of the Chrystalline humour, as likewise his Theory of the Causes of Cataracts, are fully demonstrated. To which is added for the Use of Young Students in Anatomy, the various Methods of Dissecting the Eye, whereby the Manner of Vision and the true Mechanism of the Eye are explained. By J. S., Surgeon. London. Printed for John Cooper in Fleetstreet, and Sold at the Booksellers and Pamphlet Shops of London and Westminster.

(Copy in R.C.S.) I am unable to suggest who this "J. S." was (see p. 152).

(45) LECAT. Mémoire pour servir à l'histoire des fourberies des charlatans connus sous le nom d'operateurs et des moyens de les découvrir. Précis analytique des travaux de l'Académie des Sciences de Rouen, vol. I, p. 110, 1743.

This work is quoted in full by Antonelli (77).

(46) MARTEAU. See under Dureau (80).

(47) MAUCHART, B. D. Oratio publica in D. D. Tayloris, Angli, merita Famamque habita abs Burc. David Mauchart, Med. et Chir. D. Prof. Med. Anat. et Chir. Consil. et Archiatr. Wirttb. cum Fasces Academicos Poneret Ipsis magi Calendis A. MDCCL. Tubingae apud C. H. Berger.

(Copy B.M.)

(48) MEDICAL FACULTY OF AMSTERDAM. See under Vrolick (100).

(49) MEDICAL FACULTY OF EDINBURGH. See under Scots Magazine (68).

(50) PLATNER, JO. ZACH. De motu ligamenti ciliaris. 1738. (Quoted by Hirschberg (84).)

(51) QUELMALZ. De caecitate infantum . . . . Lips. 1750. (Quoted by Hirschberg (84).)

(52) RATHLAUW, JOH. PETER. Verhandeling van de cataracta, etc. Amsterdam. 1752 (also French ed. Traité de la cataracte, etc. 1751). (Quoted by Hirschberg (84).)

II. *Lay.*

(53) ANSPACH, MARGRAVINE OF (LADY CRAVEN). Memoirs. Vol. II, p. 33. Paris. 1826.

(54) BOSWELL, JAS. Life of Johnson. Ed. G. Birkbeck Hill, p. 389. 1887.

(55) CHURCHILL, CHAS. The Ghost, Bk. iv.

(56) GIBBON. Autobiography. Ed. J. Murray, p. 36. 1896.

(57) HOGARTH, WILLIAM. See under Nichols and Steevens (86).

(58) JOHNSON, SAMUEL. See under Boswell (54), and Nichols and Steevens (86).

(59) KING, Dr WILLIAM. Political and Literary Anecdotes of his own time. Pp. 104 and 131. 2nd ed. 1819.

(60) PALMER, Dr. See under Nichols (85).

(61) WALPOLE, HORACE. Letters. Ed. Mrs Paget Toynbee, vol. III, p. 284, and vol. IV, p. 201. Oxford. 1903.

III. *Notices in Contemporary Periodical Literature.*

(62) DAILY JOURNAL, November 16th, 1736. (Quoted in Cat. Latin Prints. 2325. B.M.)

(63) GENTLEMAN'S MAGAZINE. 1736, p. 616. (Notice of attendance at Playhouse with Ward and Mrs Mapp, p. 647.) Latin epistle (see Appendix, p. 215). 1738, p. 47 (Translation of Latin epistle). 1761, p. 226 (Extract from Proposals for printing his *Travels and Adventures.* "A Masterpiece of Bombast"). 1781, p. 336 (Anecdote).

(64) THE GRUB-STREET JOURNAL. No. 293, August 7th, 1735. See Appendix, p. 210.

(65) MEDICAL ESSAYS AND OBSERVATIONS. Vol. IV, p. 383. Edinburgh. 1771. (Review of the *Treatise on the Diseases of the Chrystalline Humour of a Human Eye.* "Seems to aim at something new . . . but expresses himself in a manner that makes us suspect we may mistake his meaning.")

(66) MERCURE DE FRANCE. June 1737. (Quoted by Antonelli (77).) (Claim to cure squint "par une opération prompte, presque sans douleur, et sans crainte d'aucun accident".)

(67) ST JAMES'S EVENING POST. July 19th, 1737. (Quoted by Nichols and Steevens (86).) (Advertisement of *Epistle to a young Student.* See (75).)

(68) SCOTS MAGAZINE. 1744, p. 295. (Declaration by Roy. Coll. of Phys.); p. 322 (Poetical Essay comparing T. with Whitfield, see Appendix, p. 214); p. 344 (Announcement of his return to town). 1749, p. 252 (Notice of another tour. Arrived Edinburgh, April 19th; left for Dublin, May 16th).

IV. *Squibs and Skits.*

(69) The English Impostor detected; or, the History of the Life and Fumigation of the Renown'd Mr. J— T—, Oculist.

>Ex fumo dare lucem
>Raro antecedentem scelestem
>Deseruit pede paena Claudo.
>
>Hor.

Dublin. Printed in the Year M. DCC. XXXII.

(Copy in B.M.) For review of contents, see p. 162.

(70) A Faithful and full Account of the Surprising Life and Adventures of the Celebrated Doctor Sartorius Sinegradibus, as also of many wonderful Operations he performs in this City. Edinburgh. Printed for the Author, and sold by the Society of Running Stationers.

(Copy in B.M.) For review of contents, see p. 162.

(71) The Life and extraordinary History of the Chevalier John Taylor, Member of the most celebrated Academies, Universities and Societies of the Learned—Chevalier in several of the first Courts in the World—Illustrious (by patent) in the Apartments of many of the greatest Princes—Ophthalmiater Pontificial, Imperial and Royal—to his late Majesty—to the Pontificial Court—to the Person of Her Imperial Majesty—to the Kings of Poland, Denmark, Sweden, etc.—to the several Electors of the Holy Empire—to the Royal Infant Duke of Parma—to the Prince of Saxe-Gotha, Serenissime Brother to her Royal Highness the Princess Dowager of Wales—to the Prince Royal of Poland—to the late Prince of Orange—to the present Princes of Bavaria, Modena, Lorrain, Brunswick, Anspach, Bareith, Liege, Salzbourg, Middlebourg, Hesse-cassel, Holstein, Zerbst, Georgia, etc.—Citizen of Rome by a public Act in the name of the Senate and People—Fellow of that College of Physicians—Professor in Opticks—Doctor in Medicine and Doctor in Chirurgery in several Universities abroad. Who has been on his Travels upwards of thirty Years, with little or no Interruption, during which, he has not only been several times in every Town of these Kingdoms, but in every Kingdom, Province, State, and City of the least Consideration—in every Court—presented to every Crowned Head and Sovereign Prince in all Europe, without Exception. Containing the greatest Variety of the most entertaining and interesting Adventures that 'tis presumed has ever been published in any Language. Written from Authentic Materials, and published by his Son, John Taylor, Oculist. In two Volumes. Dublin. Printed for D. Chamberlain in Smock Alley. M, DCC, LXI.

This flamboyant title-page is, of course, an imitation of that which is prefixed to the authentic *Travels and Adventures* (19), and is, no doubt, designed to give an air of verisimilitude to the alleged authorship by the Chevalier's son.

(Copy in B.M.) For review of contents, see p. 163.

(72) A New Song. "Ye Lovers of Physick! come lend me your Ear." (Broadsheet ballad in B.M.) See Appendix, p. 217.

(73) The Operator: A Ballad Opera. London: Printed for the Author, and sold by T. Payne, Bookseller, in Round Court in the Strand, opposite York Buildings. 1740.

(Copy in B.M.) For review of contents, see p. 161.

(74) A Receipt of a ready composition on the diseases of the . . . eyes. (Quoted by Hirschberg (84, p. 297).) I have been unable to find a copy of this work.

(75) An Epistle to a young Student at Cambridge; with the Characters of the three great Quacks, Mapp, Taylor and Ward: with the methods they used to make themselves famous, etc. Beautifully printed, price 6d. (Quoted by Nichols and Steevens (86) from *St James's Evening Post*, July 19th, 1737.)

MODERN REFERENCES

(76) ANNALES D'OCULISTIQUE. Vol. cv, p. 206, 1891. (Copy of an advertisement at Rheims, 1765.)

(77) ANTONELLI, A. Arch. d'Opht., vol. XXII, p. 45, 1902. (Question of T.'s Squint operation. Quotes Lecat (45) in full.)

(78) BEER, J. Report, I, 135. (Quoted by Hirschberg (84, p. 299).)

(79) DICTIONARY OF NATIONAL BIOGRAPHY. Art. "Taylor".

(80) DUREAU. Gaz. méd. de Paris, 1891, pp. 37 and 133. (Contains Caqué's and Marteau's accounts of the Chevalier.)

(81) v. DUYSE, A. Les Oculistes ambulants à Gand au 18me Siècle. Annales de la Soc. de Méd. de Gand. 64 Année. 4. Fasc. p. 198.

(82) FRANK MORTIMER. Annals of Ophth. vol. XIV, p. 31, 1905.

(83) HENNEMANN. Ueber eine neue Reihe subcut. Operat. Rostock. 1843. (One of those who reviewed T.'s claim as discoverer of tenotomy.) (Quoted by Schrön (94).)

(84) HIRSCHBERG, J. Graefe-Saemisch Handbuch d. ges. Augenheilk. II Theil, XIV Bd. xxiii Kap. 3 Buch, II Theil, p. 289, 1909.

(85) NICHOLS, J. Literary Anecdotes of XVIII Century. Vol. II, p. 383, 1812–15; vol. VIII, pp. 400 and 410; vol. IX, p. 696. (Account of a picture of Taylor. "The Doctor is mounted in a decent Rostrum, and dressed in the same manner, and with a similar cushion before him as described in p. 400 [of vol. VIII. See p. 148]. He is holding forth to a polite and crowded audience, in which a number of physicians and others, sitting at a long table provided with pens, ink and paper, are represented as taking down his honeyed words.")

(86) NICHOLS, J. and STEEVENS, GEO. Genuine works of Wm. Hogarth, 1808. Vol. I, p. 89 (Johnson's opinion of T. Story of Prince Herculaneum,

etc.). Vol. II, p. 144 (Description of Hogarth's Consultation of Physicians);
p. 327 (Poems on T., Ward, & Mapp); p. 332 (Advertisement of *Epistle to
a young Student*).

(87) NORFOLK ARCHAEOLOGY. Vol. VIII, pp. 314 and 317, 1879.

(88) NORRIE, GORDON. Janus, vol. I, p. 227, 1896.

(89) NOTES AND QUERIES. Vol. II, vii, p. 115, vol. VII, vii, p. 82.

(90) PANSIER, P. Ann. d'Oc. vol. CXXXIV, p. 338, 1905. (T.'s claim to
have taught Daviel.)

(91) PETTIGREW, T. J. Med. Portrait Gallery. III. Life of Jas. Ware.

(92) RIBAIL. Communication through Velpeau to the Paris Academy,
September 14th, 1841. (Quoted by Schrön (94). One of the revivers of
T.'s claim to have performed a rational squint operation.)

(93) SCHMIDT'S JAHRBUCH. Vol. XXX, p. 134. (Quoted by Schrön (94).
First statement reviving T.'s claim to squint operation.)

(94) SCHRÖN, H. Arch. f. Ophth. vol. XX, i, p. 151, 1874.

(95) SMITH, J. CHALONER. British Mezzotinto Portraits, p. 429, 1883.
(Account of Riche's portrait, engraved by John Faber, Jun.) This portrait
is prefixed to the *Mechanismus des Auges* (4 and 4a).

(96) STRICKER, W. Jl. d. Chir. u. Augenh. v. Walther u. v. Ammon,
vol. XXXII (Neue Folge II), pp. 265 and 411, 1843; vol. XXXV, p. 488, 1846.

(97) TAYLOR, J. (Grandson of Chevalier). Records of My Life. 2 vols.
Vol. I, pp. 11, 13, 14, 16, 19, 20, 23, 24. London. 1832.

(98) TRUC and PANSIER. Hist. de l'Opht. à l'école de Montpellier,
pp. 224 and 274, 1907.

(99) TWISS. Life of Eldon. Vol. I, p. 321.

(100) VROLICK, G. Jl. d. Chir. u. Augenh. v. Walther u. v. Ammon,
vol. XXXIII (Neue Folge III), p. 216, 1844.

APPENDIX I

(From The Grub-Street Journal. No. 293. Thursday, August 7th, 1735)

(Page 2, col. 3.) We hear that Dr Taylor has brought with him from
Italy, a specimen of a most exquisite piece of workmanship in enamel,
intended to represent, in 385 figures, the several diseases of the globe of the
eye, (made after his own designs) which he shews to the curious that
honour him with a visit, at his house in Great Suffolk-street. 'Tis said, that
this work (which is the only of its kind yet known) from its great use to his
pupils, for instructing them in the principles of the science he professes,
gave very great satisfaction to the academies of Paris. As this gentleman
has now completely finish'd his apparatus for his curious operations of the

eyes, and is so universally known to make no secret of any part of his profession, 'tis not doubted but curiosity will bring to him from the several
parts of these kingdoms, as many spectators of distinction, and more
particularly those who are related in the faculty, as he has been honoured
with in foreign parts, it appearing that not a day pass'd but a multitude of
persons, as well of superior quality as the first of those whose education led
them to be judges, has been present on these occasions in every place he has
pass'd through; and what has added greatly to their satisfaction, has been,
that he has furnish'd their curiosity with seeing nearly 100 different operations on the eyes, amongst which there are upwards of 60 of his own,
invention; that he gives little or no pain in any of [his] operations; that
they have never any painful attendants; and that, notwithstanding the
delicacy of this sort of work, they are almost always attended with success;
all which, 'tis hop'd, at this time can admit of no doubt, after his having
been so often receiv'd for these his happy discoveries, not with respect only,
but as a member of the body of physicians in several of the most celebrated
universities abroad.

APPENDIX II

(From *A Parallel between the late celebrated Mr Pope and Dr Taylor*)

> Hail, curious Oculist! to thee belongs
> To know what secret Springs of Vision move
> The Ball of Sight; what inward cause retards
> Their Native Force; what Operation clears
> A cloudy Speck, or bids the total Frame
> Resume the lustre of the lucid Ray
> ... 'Tis thine to tell—how veiled to gloomy Shade
> The darkling Eye retires, nor feels the Force
> Of solar Beam—anon a darting Gleam
> Shoots thro' the Glass and gives the bright'ning Orb
> To visit Light—I see the Liquid stream
> Flow, as the guiding Hand directs the Way
> And bids it enter, where a total Gloom
> Had drawn dark Cover o'er the Seat of Sight,
> Whether in Choroied, or nervous Net
> Fair Vision shines,* thither the streaming Rays
> Converge their Force; and in due Order Range
> Their coloured Forms.—Anon the Patient sees
> A new Creation rising to the View
> In Living Light! There blows the flow'ry Mead
> With Sweets of every bloom, there limpid Rill
> Glides on soft Foot.—Here fair POMONA smiles

* This refers to the discussion whether the choroid or retina is the immediate
seat of vision. See his book, *An Impartial Inquiry into the Seat of the Immediate Organ
of Sight* (7).

In luxury of Charm . . . . There FLORA paints
Her vari-coloured Train.—Here Lunar Orb
Soft sheds her Silver Light to cheer the Gloom
Of languid Night, 'till Orient Sun reveals
A living Scene, with radiant Lustre spread . . . .

Go on, Thou Favourite of Heav'n, to bless
The darkling World with Light, give it to see
The Maker's Works, and teach the grateful Tongue
To sing his Praise for what the Eye beholds
To Rapture rais'd, fair Work of Power divine.
　　While others court the Populace for Fame,
And envy Merit, which they cannot claim,
Be thine the Task to beam in open Day,
And shine with Lustre of unborrow'd Ray.

APPENDIX III

(Elogium by Dr W. King. See p. 159)

HIC EST, HIC VIR EST,
Quem docti, indoctique omnes impensè mirantur,
JOHANNES TAYLOR;
Caecigenorum, caecorum & caecutientium
Quotquot sunt ubique,
Spes unica, solamen, salus.
Quorum causâ
Cunctas Europae peregravit regiones;
Neque usquam gentium fuit hospes,
Nisi in patriâ suâ.

Russicis, Suecicis, Lusitanicis,
Titulis, phaleris, torquibus
Decorus incedit:
Totoque orbe nemine cuiquam ignotus
Nisi sibi.

Orator summus non factus, sed natus,
Vocis, perinde atque manûs celeritate insignis,
Scit Latinè, Gallicè, Italicè, Germanicè fari,
Omnes callens linguas
Aequè ac sermonem patrium.

Vultu compto, corpore procero, fronte urbanâ gloriosus
Ingenioque praeditus prope singulari,
Artem amandi, et amoris remedium,
Plenius et melius Nasone ipso
Edidicit, docuit, exercuit.

Mirificus fabulator, magnificus promissor,
Rerum copiâ, artiumque varietate abundans,
Sese exhibet, effert, praedicat
In gymnasiis, in gynaeceis, in conviviis, in triviis;
Philosophando gloriam magnam adeptus,
Maximam saltando.

In peregrinis civitatibus
Equos, servosque innumeros, quos vix Satrapes
Potest habere,
Ille alit,
Domi verò,
Quae est moderatio animi sui,
Uno vili mancipio
Contentus vivit.

In celeberrimas cooptatus est Academias:
Neque tamen moribus, neque vultu, neque vestitu
Videtur Academicus.

Regnorum omnium arcana scrutari potuit:
Neque tamen speculator sagax,
Neque regis cujusquam legatus,
Neque usquam fuit vir aulicus.

Praemia, dona, permulta, amplissima accepit;
Permulta corrasit, pecuniae appetentior:
Et nondum eheu! Locupletatur.

Plures scripsit libros, quàm quivis possit legere:
Qui facinoribus tamen suis egregiis
Haud sufficiunt enumerandis.

Sexcentis primariis viris lumina reddidit
Plusquam sexcentis, sed plebiis
Sed miseris ademit.

Tum verò civibus suis praecipue colendus
Tum carminibus, docte MORELLE,* tuis celebrandus,
Tum diplomatibus honorificis, & muneribus regiis donandus;
Si Caesarem nostrum, pium, fortem, semper Augustum,
Faceret benè oculatum,
Et malos, siqui sunt, consiliarios
Tiresiâ caeciores.

I have had an opportunity since the Elogium was written of viewing our
Chevalier more nearly, and considering him with greater attention. I have
therefore been able to improve the Elogium, and add some new features to
his portrait; of which I have printed a few copies to oblige my friends.

* Qui laudes hujus ophthalmici cecinit carminibus, Graecis et Anglicanis. (I have
been unable to trace them.)

APPENDIX IV

(Elogium in the Bodleian Library, Oxford)

I am much indebted to the Librarian of the Bodleian Library for the following details. The Elogium begins:

Hic est, hic ipsus est,
Omnium numerorum et horarum homo,
Ab usque imis unguibus ad capillum summum bellissimus
Equitumque sui ordinis omnium Eques,
Auratus sit, necne, facilè princeps,
J. T.
Caecigenorum, caecorum, et caecutientium,
Quotquot sunt ubique,
Spes unica, solamen, salus.

It is in folio and extends to four pages. There is no indication of date or place of printing. Bound with it is a similar Elogium on Beau Nash, evidently from the same press. This has been catalogued by the Bodleian authorities under W. King.

APPENDIX V

(From *Scots Magazine*, 1744, p. 322)

In G. Whitfeldum et J. Taylorum

Valete, iterumque valete,
Georgi Whitfelde,
&
Johannes Taylore.

Histrionum
Par illustrissimum!
Alter oculorum sartor
Alter animorum corruptor:
Hic visûs
Ille mentis aciei
Caliginem offundens!
Ambo patriae nostrae direptores,
In hac una scilicet re,
Mercedem & nummos
Unde, unde, extricando
Simplices & ingenui;
Ambo in ruinam nati
Generis humani.
Interea, ob stultam credulitatem,
Illorum sectatores deplendi;

Et, ne quid plus detrimenti
Republica capiat,
Isti, ob insolentem audaciam,
Ad Anticyram relegandi,
Ut qui se alios curare stultè putant,
Ipsi insaniam & nequitiam deponant,
Ex patria hacce quaeso facessite,
Nunquam iterum huc redituri.
Valedictio publica vobis habita
A rei divinae & medicae
Professoribus, sit posteris
Exemplo, ne illi nimis temerè
Agyrtis & circulatoribus,
Vel sacris vel profanis,
Sese decipiendos dedant.

APPENDIX VI

(From *Gentleman's Magazine*, 1736, p. 647)

Sir,   Windsor, October 16.
    The following letter to the famous travelling Oculist, containing some Curiosity in Thought and Expression, is at your Service, for the Entertainment of your Readers.

    Domine,
    O tu, qui in oculis hominum versaris, & quamcumque tractas rem, *acu* tangis, salve!—Tu, qui instar *Phoebi*, lumen orbi, & orbes luminibus reddis, iterum salve!—
    Cum per te *Gallia*, per te nostrae *Academiae*, duo regni lumina, clarius intuentur, cur non ad urbem *Edinburgi*, cum toties & ubique *Erras*, cursum tendis? nam quaedam coecitas cives illic invasit. Ipsos magistratus *Gutta Serena* occupavit, videntur enim videre, sed nil vident.—idcirco tu istam *Scoticam Nebulam* ex oculis remove, & quodcumque latet in tenebris, in lucem profer.—Illi violenter carcerem, tu oculos leniter reclude; illi lucem *Porteio* ademerunt, tu illis lucem restitue, & quamvis fingant se *dupliciter* videre, fac, ut *simpliciter* tantum oculo irretorto conspiciant,—Peractoque cursu, ad *Angliam* redi artis tuae plenus, Toriosq: (ut vulgo vocantur) qui adhuc coecutiunt & hallucinantur, illuminatio.—Ab ipsis clericis, siqui sint coeci ductores, nubem discute; imo ipso Sole Lunaque, cum laborant eclipsi, quae, instar tui ipsius, transit per varias regiones obumbrans, istam molem caliginis amoveto.—Sic eris Sol Mundi, sic eris non solum nomine *Sartor*, sed re Oculorum omnium *Resarcitor*; sic omnis Charta Publica tuam *Claritudinem* celebrabit, & ubicunque *frontem* tuam ostendis, nemo non te, O Vir *Spectatissime*, admirabitur.—Ipse lippus scriptor hujus epistolae maxime gauderet te medicum *illustrissimum*, cum omnibus tuis oculatis testibus, *Vindsoriae* videre.—Vale.—.

(1738, p. 47.) In a subsequent number this epistle is thus rendered into
English:

> Hail, visionaire to all mankind,
> A *sight*, I mean, to all the blind;
> An eye to the *world* as Phoebus gives,
> Your art a world of eyes relieves.
> Tho' often blunders you commit,
> The mark you miss, you ever hit.
> The nation's two *dimsighted eyes*,
> Our cloudy universities,
> By you are brightened:—*France* to you
> Owes the *enlargement of her view*:
> And since a vagrant ev'rywhere
> You strole, to make all *Europe* stare
> To *Edinburgh* (why not?) repair.
> *Scotch* loons connive thro' *drop serene*
> They *seem to see* but nothing ken.
> Clear from their native mist their sight
> And works of darkness bring to light;
> Their eyelids gradually dilate;
> Not as they forc'd the prison gate,
> When Porteous they of life bereft,
> Benighted darkling, dangling left.
> To th' undiscerning magistrate
> That rules with *oversight* the state,
> For double views oblique and sly,
> Give a *direct*, a *single* eye;
> Make every *second-sighted* keeper,
> Of publick peace, a single peeper.
> This progress made, big with success
> Return; with opticks *England* bless,
> *Tories*, to sense of sight so lost,
> They knew not when they saw a *post*
> Illumin. If blind guides there be,
> Dispel the clouds that seers may see.
> The sun and moon with magic touch,
> When by eclipse extinguish'd, *couch*;
> (Wand'ring like you eclipses shed,
> Sad influence and darkness spread,)
> So shall the all-enlightening sun,
> Parent of day, and you be one,
> *Taylor* by name and sole *retailer*
> Of fresh new sight in case of failure
> In each diurnal publick paper,
> The lustre of your skill shall appear,
> And gazeing crowds shall throng the place,

Where you expose your *sightly* face
These lines (with half an eye I write)
Bright Sir, to *Windsor* you invite
Where your *eye-witnesses* and you, Sir,
I long to see: till then adieu, Sir.

RUSTIC.

APPENDIX VII

A NEW SONG

I

Ye Lovers of Physick! come lend me your Ear,
All disinterested I pray you draw near,
My Tale's of a Doctor and of a Professor
The first a skill'd man, the last an Oppressor.
Down; down—down, dery, down.

II

Our worthy *Professor* (whom few can excel)
Is a Spreader of Calumny, greedy as Hell,
His principal Study is hoarding of *Pelf,*
And ne'er does an Action but tends to himself.
Dery down.

III

This *Gown-man* so noted, by silly mean Lies
Attacked here a Stranger for curing of *Eyes,*
A Subject on which he himself ne'er spake Sense
Though he *lectur'd* on't yearly for gaining of Pence.
Dery down.

IV

He began on the Doctor's Arrival to smell,
(For joined with his Greed he is cunning and fell)
That a Rival so bright, who no Secret did hide,
Might quickly eclipse a few Grains of his Pride.
Dery down.

V

To ward of this Blow, from Morning to Night,
Thus accosted his *Mates,* "and said it was right
"To discourage a man of such Learning and Parts,
"Because prejudicial to *Masters of Arts.*
Dery down.

VI

"You know he can teach, when our Students have Clink,
"But those of toom Pockets can't learn, (as we think)
"If they want but a Shilling of our common Fee
"We send them a-packing, to our *Class* they're not free.
Dery down.

VII

"Ye cannot forget, ev'n a Friend of our own,
"A Brother by Trade, well skill'd, of Renown,
"Was debarr'd a Dissection, he intended to make
"At my *Instigation*, lest my Trade it should break.
Dery down.

VIII

"Is it fair that a Stranger go off with our Wealth?
"Let the Blind and Blear-ey'd be deprived of their Health
"Far rather, than that it shou'd ever be said,
"That our College, so famous, wants Skill in the Trade.
Dery down.

IX

"Our *Noble Infirmary*, built at great Cost,
"By the Bounty of those who love the Poor most
"Shall never be fill'd for their Use, by this *Man*,
"For there shall I swagger, let 'em do what they can."
Dery down.

X

And thus our Professor, possess'd with Envy,
Spread Stories about, of this and that Eye
As hurt by the Doctor, who truly did cure;
Beware then, my Friends, of what comes from his Lure.
Dery down.

XI

But great Doctor Taylor thou neat-handed Man,
Judge not of this Nation by this single one,
For those of the College who do you oppose,
Are but such the Professor can lead by the Nose.
Dery down.

XII

Let those do their best by *Libels* in Print,
The Men of sound Sense will *ne'er take the Hint*
To condemn you at Random, not knowing yo . . .
They'll leave that to the College, those Wits of . . . .
Dery down.

XIII

Much more cou'd I say, as the helpless do groan,
Depriv'd of their *House* that's truly their own,
What Grudge must the *Donors* retain in their Breast
To see it lock'd up, and the Poor thus opprest.
                              Dery down.

XIV

But the rest I'll refer 'till the *Doctor* is gone,
Then with Grief and with Tears we'll be making our Moan
When none of the *Faculty* dare use the *Needle*
Tho' they Strutted thro' *France*, and there danc'd to a Fiddle.
                              Dery down.

APPENDIX VIII

(Latin verses beneath Taylor's portrait in *Mechanismus des Auges*)

Effigiem Taylor, tibi qui demissus ab alto est
    Turba alias expers luminis, ecce vides
Hic maculas tollit, cataractas deprimit omnes,
    Amissum Splendens excitat ille jubar.
Mirandâ praxi sublata ophthalmia, quaevis
    Artifici dextra gutta serena cadit.
Ecce virum cujus cingantur tempora lauro;
    Dignum qui laudes saecula longa canant.

(Other verses from his works)

Taylorus promptam caecis afferre salutem
    Gnarus, quo vadet, luminis instar erit.
At Basilea tuis medicis nunc junctus in aevum
    Omne choro medico sideris instar eris.

CHAPTER X

Historical Notes*

BY GEORGE COATS

THE CHEVALIER TAYLOR'S SON

FOR good and for ill, the son of the Chevalier Taylor was
but the shadow of his more illustrious father. His respectable stay-at-home existence pales into insignificance beside
the Chevalier's meteoric career; yet a brief account of the man
and of his sole contribution to literature may still possess a
certain interest.

John Taylor, Junior, the Chevalier's only son, was born in
1724, in the twenty-first year of his father's age (26).† While still
a boy he was sent to Paris, where for five years he studied French
and the classics at the Collège du Plessis. Returning to London
"about his fifteenth year" he lived for a while with his mother,
and on the return of his father, in 1742, from a triumphal progress through Spain and Portugal, he began to study the rudi-
ments of his art under the tuition of that able preceptor. Probably
the restless wanderings of his father soon left him in an independent or semi-independent position; in 1753 he speaks of
having had "experience of his own for nine years successively in
London"; at any rate, in 1747 or 1749 the Chevalier departed on
a prolonged continental tour, and left him to his own devices.

At an early age he fell in love with the daughter of a respectable
tradesman, a lady who, according to the testimony of her son,
was sprightly, intelligent, good humoured, fond of literature,
and conversant with history. Her father, however, objected to

* Published in the *Royal London Ophthalmic Hospital Reports*, vol. XX, p. 129,
March 1916.
† This fact may be added to the evidence that the date 1708 which is sometimes
given as that of the Chevalier's birth is erroneous (*R.L.O.H. Reports*, vol. XX, p. 2).

the match, and the lovers were therefore obliged to conduct their courtship by means of secret meetings at Bedlam, which at that time was a kind of public show, open to casual visitors on payment of a penny or twopence.* Despite, or in consequence of, these impediments, however, the marriage took place. Practice must also have been prosperous at this time, for in addition to a house in Hatton Garden, where Taylor carried on his profession, we hear of a cottage at Highgate, with two female servants, one foot-boy, and a chaise. The regular yearly advent of an addition to the family, however, necessitated a retrenchment of these exuberances; the cottage was relinquished, and from this period till his death, at the age of sixty-three, he became wholly settled at Hatton Garden. Here, if there be truth in obituary notices, he became "highly distinguished in his profession as an oculist"(2); here his father, during his infrequent visits to London, sought refreshment, saw patients, and contributed counsel from the vast storehouse of his experience; here, after his death, two of his sons carried on the family vocation in the third generation.

The first of Taylor's great patients was the Duke of Ancaster, to whose seat in Lincolnshire he was twice summoned, and whom he cured of a violent inflammation of the eyes(1). The Duke esteemed him also as a companion, and sometimes invited him to spend his Christmas holidays in the country. He bestirred himself also in 1772, on the death of the Chevalier, to obtain for him the post of Oculist to George III, and almost succeeded, but the superior influence of the Duke of Bedford, who had been successfully operated upon by the Baron Wenzel, procured the office for that celebrated man(26).

Through the influence of his friend, Dr Monsey, Taylor was also called upon to treat the Earl of Godolphin, who was so much

* "To my great surprise I found a hundred people at least, who having paid their twopence apiece, were suffered unattended to run rioting up and down the wards making sport of the miserable inhabitants. I saw them in a loud laugh of triumph at the ravings they had occasioned", *The World*, June 7th, 1753. Quoted by Crocker, *Boswell's Life of Johnson*, year 1775. Boswell and Johnson paid a visit to the asylum.

charmed with the manner in which he bled him—his Grace being very fat—that he afterwards insisted on retaining his services even in other than ocular affections. Cheselden is said also to have been one of his patrons, and frequently to have sent him patients.

The year 1753 saw the first public formulation of a scheme which Taylor afterwards laboured in vain to fulfil. His private benevolence, it appears, had brought him into difficulties. By public advertisements he had offered gratuitous assistance to all the poor who laboured under infirmities of the eyes, and he had even supplied them with such medicines as their cases might require. Not unnaturally these charitable activities soon involved him in a "vast expense", and led to a proposal for the founding of a hospital for the blind. The institution was not to be purely eleemosynary. Its eminent patrons, the Duke of Ancaster and the Right Hon. the Earl of Godolphin, admitted the justice of appropriating "some reasonable salary for the Encouragement of his Deserts, who first open'd this laudable Scheme". Unfortunately the public failed to rise to the height of its opportunity. No hospital was founded, and Taylor was forced to devise a modified plan whereby all subscribers of the trifling sum of two guineas might send poor patients to his house at Hatton Garden. The same offer, made to the "several parishes of the metropolis", met with "but small countenance" (1, 2, 26).

The possibilities of this scheme did not escape the keen eye of the Chevalier, who gives it his blessing in his Autobiography, and offers to share the labours, and no doubt the recompense, of the good work (4). Along with the advertisements of "Jesuit drops", "Elixir of Bardana" and other quack remedies, there appears in the *Public Advertiser* of December 5th, 1761, an invitation to all sufferers from diseases of the eye "to attend the Chevalier henceforward, at his Son's in Hatton Garden, where every morning before Ten, the Poor may, as in former Times, have his best Assistance, and where Subscriptions are taken in, with Promise of mutual Care, agreeable to an Advertisement so often addressed by the Son to the Nobility for that End".

It is difficult to adjudicate on the disinterestedness or otherwise of the younger Taylor's part in these transactions. The Chevalier's so-called gratuitous treatment at Hatton Garden is savagely attacked as a mere fraudulent device in the *Operator* (1740, see p. 32), but on the other hand the writer of the son's obituary notice in the *Gentleman's Magazine*(2) states that he continued his beneficence in spite of the discouraging response of the public, and compares his philanthropy with that of a Hanway or a Howard.

The ostentatious manner in which Taylor advertised his scheme and pushed his claims in connexion therewith, as well as the laudatory letters which he inserts in his published work, have a suspicious appearance to a modern eye, but care should be taken not to apply the ethical standard of the twentieth century to transactions of the eighteenth. Duddell, for instance, whom no one accuses of being a quack, never hesitated to give the names and addresses of those upon whom he had performed cures.

According to his son, Taylor was a good French and Latin scholar and universally respected in private life for his integrity(26). He was fond of the drama, and the house in Hatton Garden was a resort of some of the most celebrated actors of the day. If the following tale be true, the connexion was not without its utilitarian aspect:

"Garrick was once present when my father was going to perform an operation on the cataract; and though the patient was timid and fearful, he was entertained so much by Garrick's humour that he underwent the operation with great fortitude and was rewarded by its success".

Poetry also, in the person of a certain Mr Boyce, paid its admiring tribute(1):

> While modest Merit does its rays conceal,
> Let the just Muse draw the injurious Veil,
>
> .   .   .   .   .   .
>
> No longer timid in Retirement pine,
> But claim the Notice that is justly Thine.

Say, of the Blessings to Mankind decreed,
From great Hippocrates to greater Mead . . .
Can any with thy noble Science Vie
Which guards the guiding Lamp of Life, the Eye?
        Etc., etc.

In the meridian of his life Taylor was distinguished by the "vivacity of his humour" and his quickness in repartee. In his later years, however, over-confidence in certain false friends led him into pecuniary difficulties, and overclouded the cheerfulness of his disposition. His most intimate friend was William Oldys,* the famous antiquarian, biographer and bibliographer. The old scholar had his share of the peculiarities of his tribe. When he passed an evening at Hatton Garden he preferred the kitchen fireside, lest he should meet any of the other visitors. He could not smoke his pipe with ease till his chair was set close to a particular crack in the floor. His shyness led him to refuse an introduction to the gorgeous Chevalier, but one evening that great man invaded his retreat, and addressing him in Latin kept up a colloquy for two hours, whilst the admiring son, conscious of his inferiority as a scholar, interposed an occasional remark. This

---

* Born in 1696. In 1731 he came under the patronage of Harley, Earl of Oxford, and in 1738 was appointed his Literary Secretary. He was associated with Johnson in preparing a *catalogue raisonnée* of Harley's books, and also arranged and catalogued the famous Harleian Miscellany. He rendered a real service to biography by his rebellion against the florid and unveracious style into which it had fallen during the seventeenth century. His irregular habits brought him to the Fleet prison for debt, but after two years he was released by the Duke of Norfolk and given the post of Norroy King of Arms in the Herald's office. Occasionally his severer studies were diversified by flights into an airier region. He confessed to being the author of an "Anacreontick", beginning:
        "Busy, curious, thirsty fly!"
in which that insect is humanely invited to share his cup, or even, should it feel equal to the feat, to drink the whole of it. He was also responsible for the following play upon his own name:
        "In word and *Will I am* a friend to you,
          And one friend *Old is* worth a hundred new".
He died in 1761, and Taylor, as the principal creditor, defrayed his funeral expenses and obtained possession of his books. (See a Memoir by J. Yeowell in *Notes and Queries*, ser. III, vol. I, 1862.)

tale is told by the Chevalier's grandson in refutation of the strictures of Johnson, "that literary hippopotamus", on his grandfather's Latinity (see *R.L.O.H. Reports*, vol. xx, p. 31); in reality, Johnson was envious because Taylor excelled him in the colloquial use of Latin (26).

In 1753, Oldys, in collaboration with his friend, published his *Observations on the Cure of William Taylor, the Blind Boy of Ightham, in Kent*, etc.; but the contents of this work will be considered more appropriately in the second section of these notes.

SOME EARLY OBSERVATIONS ON RESTORATION OF SIGHT IN THE CONGENITALLY BLIND

In speculating on the sensations of a man born blind and restored to sight, scientific observers were anticipated by philosophers and philosophers by practical men of affairs.

No doubt the earliest observation bearing on the subject is that of the blind man (Mark viii. 22–6) who at first saw "men as trees walking", and only after a second application of the divine power "saw every man clearly". In more modern times the first reference to the subject which I have been able to find dates from 1528, and is contained in Sir Thomas More's *Dialogue* "Of the Veneracion and Worship of Ymages and Relyques" (6). I may perhaps be pardoned for transcribing the passage in full.

As I remēber me that I have hard my father tell of a begger, that in kyng Hēry his daies the first, cam w^{h} his wife to saint Albonis. And there was walking about the towne begging a five or six dayes before the kinges commynge thither, saienge y^{t} he was borne blinde, and never sawe in hys lyfe. And was warned in hys dreame that he shoulde come out of Berwyke, where he said he had euer dwelled, to seke Saynt Albon, & that he had ben at his shryne & had not been holpen. And therefore he woulde go seke hym at some other place for he had hard some say sins he came y^{t} sainct Albonys body shold be at Colon, and in dede such a contencion hath ther ben. But of troth as I am surely informed, he lieth here at saint Albonis, sauing some reliques of him, which thei there show shrined. But to tell you forth whan ye kynge was comen, and the towne full, sodaynelye this blind man, at saint Albonis shrine had his sight agayne, and a myracle solemply rongen, and *te deum* songen, so that nothyng was talked of in al the towne, but this myracle. So happened it than, that duke Humfry of glocester* a great wise man and very wel lerned, hauing great Joy to se such a myracle, called ye pore man unto hym. And first shewing him self Joyouse of goddes glory so shewed in the gettinge of his sight, & exortinge hym to mekeness, & to none ascribing of any part of the worship to him self nor to be proude of the peoples prayse, which would call him a good & a godly man thereby. At last he loked well upon his eyen, and asked whyther he could neuer se nothing at al, in al his life before. And whan as well his wyfe as him self affermed fastely no, thā he loked aduisedly upō his eien again, & said, I beleue you very wel, for me thinketh that ye cañot se well yet. "Yes syr", quoth he, "I thanke god and his holy marter, I can see nowe as well as any man." "Ye can", quoth the duke, "what colour is my gowne?" thā anone the begger tolde him. "What colour", quoth he, "is this mans gowne": he told him also, & so forth without any sticking he told the names of al ye colours that coulde bee shewed him. And whan my lord saw y^t he had him walke faytoure,†

> "Eftsoones the Gard, which on his state did wait,
> Attacht that faytor false, and bound him strait".
> *Faerie Queene*, I, xii, 35.

& made him be set openly in the stockes. For though he could haue sene soudēly by miracle ye difference betwene diuers colours, yet coulde he not by the syght so sodenly tell the names of all these colours, but if he had knowē them before, no more than the names of al the men y^t he should sodēly se.

Shakespeare has used an expanded version of this tale in the second part of *Henry VI* (Act II, Sc. 1)‡ adding a lameness which was cured by whipping. "If thou hadst been born blind", says Duke Humphrey to the impostor, "thou mightst as well have known all our names as thus to name the several colours we

---

* Humphrey, Duke of Gloucester, b. 1391, d. 1447, fourth son of Henry IV and uncle of Henry VI. An ambitious and unprincipled man, but a great patron of letters and collector of books.

† Faytoure = impostor, cheat.

‡ This passage is erroneously quoted by Hirschberg as the original authority for the story.

do wear. Sight may distinguish of colours; but suddenly to nominate them all, it is impossible."

Towards the end of the seventeenth century the problem was transferred to the realms of philosophical speculation, and became a subject of disputation between the Empiricists, who maintained that intellectual conceptions are derived ultimately from impressions of the senses, and the Nativists, who believed that certain ideas are not the result of experience, but are innate or inherent in the human mind. The empiricist philosophy required, of course, that the healed blind man should be unable to recognise objects by sight till he had verified their nature by his tactile or other senses; the Nativists asserted the possibility at least, that his innate ideas would give him some guidance in forming a judgment; and as neither side could appeal to any actual observations, the materials were to hand of a very pretty controversy.

The question was first raised by W. Molyneux in a letter to Locke, which is quoted in the *Essay concerning the Human Understanding*(8):

"Suppose a man born blind, and now adult, and taught by his touch to distinguish between a cube and a sphere of the same metal, and nighly of the same bigness, so as to tell, when he felt one and the other, which is the cube, which the sphere. Suppose, then, the cube and sphere placed on a table, and the blind man be made to see: quare, whether by his sight, before he touched them, he could now distinguish and tell which is the globe, which the cube?" To which the acute and judicious proposer answers, "Not. For though he has obtained the experience of how a globe, how a cube affects his touch, yet he has not yet obtained the experience, that what affects his touch so or so, must affect his sight so or so; or that a protuberant angle in the cube, that pressed his hand unequally, shall appear to his eye as it does in the cube". I agree with this thinking gentleman, etc.

In his *New Theory of Vision* (1709) Bishop Berkeley(9) devotes considerable space to an examination of the subject, and concludes, in agreement with Locke, that the cured blind man "would not consider the ideas of sight . . . as having any connection with the ideas of touch", and that "no idea entering by the eye would have a perceivable connection with the ideas to which the names earth, man, head, foot, etc., were annexed". He thought that "the sun and stars, the remotest objects as well as the nearer, would all seem to be in his eye, or rather in his mind".

The subsequent course of the controversy has been sufficiently sketched by Hirschberg(16), and need not detain us here. The weight of authority, headed by Leibnitz, appears to have been opposed to the Molyneux-Locke solution, the general line of argument being, that the blind man, considering the cube and the sphere, would reason with himself that the object which seemed alike all over would be the same as that which felt alike all over, and the object which seemed not uniform would be the one which felt irregular. This view was supported by a certain Dr Sanderson, "the greatest blind philosopher that ever was"(15).

When the matter came to be put to the proof of actual observation it was found that the conditions predicated in these speculations—a totally blind man suddenly restored to perfect sight—were in practice unattainable. For no one can be cured who is previously utterly ignorant of visual sensations; and even the most successful removal of congenital cataract has been shown to be followed by a period during which the functions of the retina remain in abeyance, the patient for the time being deriving little benefit from the operation. Moreover, the later the operation the more amblyopic the eye, so that if the cure be undertaken when the patient is old enough to analyse and describe his sensations only a very low degree of vision is to be expected.* Nevertheless, the main thesis of the Empiricists— that the man restored to sight is unable to distinguish one object from another, and that the new sense must be learned step by step, like a foreign language—has been amply substantiated.

The first contribution founded on actual observation displays

* See a recent record of a case and analysis of the literature by Augustein (*Klin. Monatsbl. f. Augen.* LII, ii, 1913, p. 521).

too evidently the cloven hoof of the journalist in search of copy, and is wholly devoid of scientific value(10). The patient, a young man aged 20, was operated upon by Roger Grant,* at Newington Butts, in Surrey, in June 1709. There was a numerous attendance of his acquaintances and friends, including "a young gentlewoman for whom he had a passion", and the minister, the Rev. Mr Caswell (or Taswell), imposed silence in order that the dawning of the new sense might be observed unperturbed by the recognition of familiar voices. Immediately after the operation "there appeared such an ecstasy in his action, that he seemed ready to swoon away in the surprise of joy and wonder". This was too much for his mother, who fell on his neck, exclaiming "My son! my son!" The lad could barely articulate, "Oh me! are you my mother?" before he fainted, whereupon the young gentlewoman—her name was Lydia—"shrieked in the loudest manner". On his recovery he exclaimed, "Is this seeing? Were you always thus happy when you said you were glad to see each other?" He offered to move, but seemed afraid of everything round him; he thought the instruments in the surgeon's hands were part of the hands themselves. After a bandage had been applied for a week, during which he attempted "to speak [in perplexed terms of his own making] of what he had in that short time observed", the young gentlewoman was deputed to unbind his eyes "as well to endear herself to him by such a circumstance, as to moderate his ecstasies by the persuasion of a voice, which had so much power over him". Before doing so, however, she solemnly warned him that he would "find there is such a thing as beauty, which may ensnare you into a thousand passions of which you now are innocent, and take you from me for ever". To which the young man passionately replied, "Dear Lydia, if I am to lose by sight the soft pantings which I have always felt when I heard your voice ... pull out these eyes, before they lead me to be ungrateful to you ... I wished for them but to see you; pull them out, if they are to make me

* See the third section of these notes.

forget you". Lydia, it is pleasing to note, "was extremely satisfied with these assurances".

Unfortunately for such slender credence as one might be disposed to grant to this highly seasoned narration, there exists
another account which puts a totally different complexion on the
affair(11). It is entitled: *A Full and True Account of a Miraculous
Cure, of a Young Man in Newington, that was Born Blind, and was
in Five Minutes brought to Perfect Sight. By Roger Grant, Oculist,*
etc. According to this pamphlet, which is written not by Grant,
but by some enemy of his, the lad was not blind, but could
recognise people, and had been seen to play at tops with other
boys. He had a speck on the "outward coat" of his left eye
which came before the pupil when he looked down, and hence
in walking he always went "with his chin on his bosom"; but
he could see objects above him, and could follow the flight of a
hawk. After the operation he came with his mother to Mr Taswell, the minister, bringing for signature a certificate couched in
the following terms:

As it would be no less Disrespectful than Injurious to the Publick,
to conceal the Merits of Mr *Roger Grant*, Oculist: Therefore We, the
Minister and Church-Wardens and Overseers of the Poor of the
Parish of *St Mary-Newington-Butts*, do certify, that *William Jones* of
the same parish, aged 20 years, who was born Blind, on his Application to Mr *Grant* aforesaid, was by him Couch'd on *Wednesday* the
19th of *June* last, and by the Blessing of God on the skilful hand of
Mr *Grant*, the said Jones in 5 minutes time was brought to see; and at
this time hath his Sight very well; this Cure being so particularly
remarkable, and performed *Gratis* by Mr *Grant*; We do therefore
give this Publick Testimony under our Hands this 25th Day of July
1709.

The minister refused to sign till the churchwardens had done
so, saying that he was satisfied neither that the lad was born blind
nor that he now saw well. In spite of the mother's tearful plea
that the gratuitousness of Grant's treatment was conditional on
the production of the certificate, and that without it a certain
eye-water essential to the completion of the cure would be with-

held, the wardens, of whom one was an expert surgeon, were equally obdurate. Finding her importunities vain, the mother now had recourse to plain forgery, and the certificate was published by Grant in the form of an advertisement in the *Daily Courant*(12) and the *British Apollo*(13). The minister refused to be drawn into a public wrangle, but warned all enquirers that he had never seen Grant in his life, had never signed a certificate, was not present at the operation, and knew nothing of it till a month later. To this repudiation Grant replied by publishing an affidavit made by the mother before Sir John Houblon, a magistrate, to the effect that by the blessing of God Grant had restored her son to sight "in five minutes"(12, 13, 19). In a similar affidavit the lad himself swears that he can see "the sand run in a glass, or any thing in common".

The impression conveyed by the whole transaction is that Grant in his ignorance, and perhaps owing to his monocular vision, attempted to couch a case of corneal opacity, and afterwards, with the effrontery which is an essential part of the outfit of the quack, sought to make capital out of his mistake.

The first observation which bears any stamp of scientific precision is the famous and often quoted description of Cheselden dating from 1728(14).* Before operation the patient had perception of light and with good illumination could distinguish colours, though afterwards he did not recognise them with certainty as the same. He was couched when between 13 and 14 years of age. At first he had no judgment of distances but thought all objects touched his eyes as those which he felt did his skin. "He knew not the Shape of any Thing, nor any one Thing from another, however different in Shape or Magnitude." "Having often forgot which was the cat and which the dog, he was ashamed to ask; but catching the cat (which he knew by feeling) he was observed to look at her steadfastly, and then

---

* Hirschberg's statement that this case is reprinted in full in the *Tatler* (No. 55) is erroneous. The *Tatler* was defunct before 1728. It is Grant's case which is there described.

setting her down, said, 'So Puss! I shall know you another time'." He was surprised that those things which he liked best did not appear most agreeable to his eyes. Two months after the operation he discovered that pictures represented solid bodies; previously he had considered them to be merely "surfaces diversified with variety of Paint". He was much surprised that they did not feel like solid bodies, and asked which was the lying sense, Feeling or Seeing. On seeing a miniature he was astonished "that a large face could be express'd in so little room". At first "he could bear but very little sight, and the things he saw he thought extremely large". When the second eye was couched objects at first appeared large to it, but not so much so as in the case of the other. He thought scarlet the most beautiful colour, but black "gave him great uneasiness". However, he became reconciled to it, but some time afterwards seeing a Negro woman "he was struck with great Horror at the Sight".

In another paper, quoted by Smith(15), Cheselden adds his experience of other cases. "They all had this in common, that having never had occasion to move their eyes, they knew not how to do it; and at first could not at all direct them to a particular object; but in time they acquired that faculty, though by slow degrees."

Oldys's account (1753) of the blind boy of Ightham cured by Taylor is greatly inferior to Cheselden's, yet not without a certain interest(1). It is entitled: *Observations on the Cure of William Taylor, the Blind Boy of Ightham, in Kent; Who being born with Cataracts in both Eyes, was at Eight Years of Age, brought to Sight on the 8th of October,* 1751, *By Mr John Taylor, Junr., Oculist, in Hatton Garden,* etc. By way of preface there is a list of noble and eminent patrons, ranging from the Duke of Ancaster to plain "Mr Froling Hogmagog", and Mr Foot an apothecary. Then follows a dedicatory epistle to Dr Monsey of Chelsea Hospital, "a singular Friend to Mr Taylor", inviting his testimony concerning that gentleman's character and abilities; to which Dr Monsey returns a gracious reply, and thus en-

PLATE IX

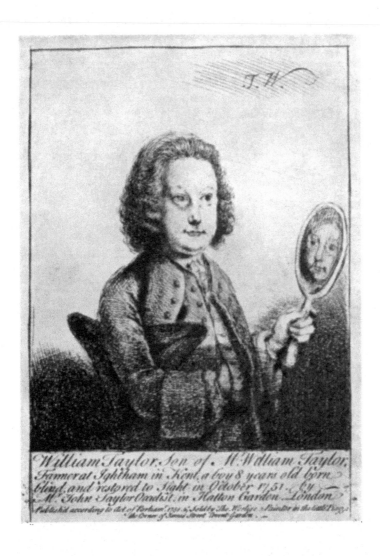

Reproduced from Royal London Ophthalmic Hospital Reports. Vol. xx.

couraged the author ventures to bring to his notice the merits of the Hospital scheme.

The treatise itself begins with a delineation of the pitiable state of the blind, and a defence of specialism in diseases of the eye. Livings are made by the curing of corns, why not by the curing of eyes? Taylor's qualifications and the Hospital scheme receive a second eulogy, and so we come to business. Before operation the boy could distinguish light from darkness. Couching was performed at his father's house, in the presence of sixteen neighbours. Taylor wished to tie him down, "but he, as he could see no danger, felt no fear", and "lay with his hands in his Pockets, till the Obstruction in his Right Eye, was, in little more than a minute, entirely removed". Asked what he saw, he answered "with a kind of mild Transport and Wonder at the strange Shapes, Forms and Colours of many Things, so incomprehensible about him, that he beheld the Room full of Lights and Moons". At the first dressing, according to the father's testimony, he saw "the Pewter on the Shelf, with the Clock and its Case", which he knew before by feeling. Oldys suspects, however, that this must have been merely an affirmative response to the leading question "Do you see the Pewter, etc.?" Soon afterwards he was delighted to see himself in a looking-glass. When he saw any large piece of furniture he was afraid to move till he was told what it was, and how far off, yet he climbed out on the gutter at the top of the house "to catch the Moon, not being apprehensive of Danger and having no notion of distances". For the latter reason also he had difficulty in picking up coins from the table. It seemed to Oldys, after the operation, that the eye was "more infantine", as if it belonged to a younger person, and was not so "strong, bold and ample in the pupil" as it would have been had it been longer exercised in the reception of images.

A certain Mr King, a Lecturer in Optics, had a theory that a blind person restored to sight would see objects inverted, and maintained that his views were established by observations on

the boy at Ightham. In this contention he received the support
of Dr Monsey, in the following terms: "The principal observation I made upon the Ightham Boy, was his confirming the
Phenomenon of Vision, of Objects being painted, inverted upon
the Retina; for when a Pin was held upright before him, he constantly directed his finger to the Head, instead of the Point, and
so *vice versâ*: How the mind turns it afterwards, is a Question of
another kind, and very hard to be resolv'd". Oldys's attitude is
cautiously sceptical. Were the boy's errors not due rather to his
ignorance of higher, lower, right and left? And is it credible that
one who at first saw objects inverted should by any amount of
practice be able subsequently to see them in an exactly opposite
manner? Yet the possibility of inverted vision is not summarily
to be rejected; with a convex glass the image is erect at one
distance, inverted at another; may not something analogous
occur in the eye owing to an insufficiency in one of the humours,
or to some irregularity in the retina or one of the other "mediums
to the sensory in the brain"? Nay, let us take heed lest we fall
into impiety. Scripture informs us that the blind man "saw
men like trees walking"; may not this mean that he saw them
with their legs in the air, like branches, and their heads on the
ground like roots?

The treatise ends, as is common in eighteenth-century pamphlets, with the names, addresses, and a brief *résumé* of the
symptoms of patients upon whom Taylor had performed
remarkable cures.

This case evidently made some stir. A print, here reproduced,
of the boy, executed by Thomas Worlige, exists in the British
Museum(s). He holds a three-cornered hat under his arm. The
left eye is depicted as normal. In the right there is an attempt to
represent a cataract; the iris and pupil are unshaded, and the eye
deviates upwards and inwards. He is holding a mirror so as to
exhibit his reflection to the spectator, but is not looking into it.

Beyond this point it is not my intention to carry the subject.
The purpose of these notes is to supplement and add some

additional cases to Hirschberg's(16) necessarily condensed account, which contains only a passing reference to Grant's case and omits Taylor's. For the further history of the subject the reader is referred to the well-known work of that author.

ROGER GRANT

The date of Roger Grant's birth is unknown; he died about 1724. According to his enemy, the writer of the *Full and True Account*(11) analysed at p. 230 of these notes, he was bred a cobbler, or, as some say, a tinker. He was a powerful Anabaptist preacher, and is said to have used his influence over his auditors to foster a belief in his semi-miraculous powers of healing. According to a more charitable view, however, he "seems to have been more ingenious and reputable than most of his brother and sister oculists; but if we may judge by his numerous advertisements he was not less vain or less indelicate". In the reign of Queen Anne he began to practise as an oculist at Mouse Alley, Wapping, and in 1710 was sworn Oculist and Operator in ordinary to the Queen. After the death of Sir William Read, in 1715, he held the same post under George I. Eighteenth-century royalty seems to have been peculiarly unfortunate in its oculists. Grant was honoured by two somewhat inconsistent notices in the *Spectator*(17). In the first he is referred to as "a Doctor in *Mouse Alley*, near Wapping, who sets up for curing cataracts upon the Credit of having, as his Bill sets forth, lost an eye in the Emperor's Service. His Patients come in upon this, and he shows the Muster-Roll, which confirms that he was in his Imperial Majesty's Troops; and he puts out their Eyes with great Success". In the second, a correspondent under the pseudonym "Philanthropus" says: "I myself have been cured by him of a Weakness of the Eyes next to Blindness, and am ready to believe anything that is reported of his Ability this Way; and know that many, who could not purchase his Assistance with money, have enjoy'd it from his Charity".

Grant's advertisements appeared twice a week with great regularity in the *British Apollo*(19), and occasionally also in other journals. They take the form sometimes of lists of patients recently cured, with their full names and addresses; sometimes of certificates similar to that which has already been quoted, signed either by the patient himself, by the minister and churchwardens, or by the mayor and aldermen of various townships throughout the country. Evidently, like other oculists of the time, he made occasional provincial tours. In the British Museum also there is a folio sheet presumably intended for distribution to the public(18): *An Account of some Cures (well attested by undeniable certificates) performed by Roger Grant, Oculist in Ordinary to his present Majesty King George, who was also Oculist to the late Queen, may be advised with every Day at his House, St Christopher's Church-yard, in Threadneedle Street,* London; from 9 in the morning till 12, in all Distempers relating to the eyes, but in no other.* This is a collection of certificates and testimonies of the usual type. It contains a graphic account of how a certain Thomas Prosar had one eye "Chouched by a great Pretender", with the result that it "perished in his head"; he remained in this miserable condition till one day Mr Grant, riding by the gate where he begged for alms, "dismounted from his horse, and in a minute's time chouched my eye, and brought me to Sight without demanding any Satisfaction". The Newington cure of course appears, and it is claimed that thirty-two other blind-born persons, as well as several cases of gutta serena, had been healed.

THE CHEVALIER TAYLOR'S GRANDSON

The birth of John Taylor, tertius, at the cottage in Highgate in 1755, moved the poet Derrick, a friend of the family, to a natal ode which commences thus:

> Muse, give Dr Taylor joy,
> For Dr Taylor has a boy,

---

* A comparison of dates seems to show that he practised simultaneously here and in Wapping.

but unfortunately fails to sustain the promise of so brilliant an opening.

He was the eldest son of his father, and after receiving his education in academies at Ponders End and in Cross Street near Hatton Garden, he was offered a post without the usual premium of £1000 as an indentured clerk in the legal office of Mr Crespigny, a King's Proctor and member of Parliament(26). The offer, however, was declined, as his father could not support him during his apprenticeship and required his assistance in his profession. In one of his title-pages the subject of the present note claims to be, like his grandfather, a graduate of the University of Basle, as well as a "Member of the Helvetic Physico-Medical Society; the Corporation of the Surgeons of London", etc., etc.(20), but concerning his medical studies the only information which he vouchsafes in his autobiography is that he attended the lectures of William Hunter at the same time as Gibbon and Adam Smith, and that the historian used to thank the lecturer courteously at the end of each meeting. He states also that he practised general surgery for many years, but always paid special attention to the eyes.

After his father's death in 1787 he carried on the profession of an oculist along with his brother Jeremiah at Hatton Garden. In 1789 he was appointed Oculist to the Prince of Wales; on the death of the Baron Wenzel he became, conjointly with his brother and through the influence of the Earl of Salisbury, Oculist to George III, and on the accession of George IV (1820) he retained the appointment. In a pecuniary sense, however, these were barren honours, and accordingly as early as 1790 he began to dally with literature, hoping to find therein a more royal road to independence than ophthalmology could offer(26). Henceforward his profession bulked less and less in his life, and he seems to indicate that before 1811 he had quite given up practice(24).

The branches of the literary calling which specially attracted him were journalism and poetry. For fifty years he was connected with the press, sometimes gratuitously, sometimes at a salary, latterly as part and afterwards sole proprietor of the *Sun* and *True Briton* newspapers. The *Sun* was founded under the auspices of Pitt, of whom he was an enthusiastic admirer, and in whose honour he composed a birthday ode annually for over twenty years. For two years also he was editor of the *Morning Post*, but the chief proprietor considered that he had "not devil enough for the conduct of a public journal". Yet he seems to have done his best to supply that deficiency by regaling certain boon companions in his office with a liberal supply of punch while waiting for the paper to go to press. Owing to the treachery of a business partner he fell into pecuniary difficulties towards the end of his life, and this led to the writing of his autobiography and to the publication of his collected poems by subscription. He died in 1831 or 1832. He was twice married, the first time in 1788, and had at least one son, who seems to have deserted finally the hereditary profession.

Some glimpses of Taylor's personality may be gathered from a review, in the *Gentleman's Magazine*, of his autobiography, the *Records of my Life*, which was published posthumously in 1832 (27). "Few men", we are told, "have lived so constantly in the eye of the metropolis." To dine frequently with men of note was not only his amusement but his interest. He had an inexhaustible stream of pleasantry and puns. "He was by nature a ready man, of bright parts, and perhaps too volatile for profound study. Conversation was therefore his library in a great degree ... what he could gather was always on the surface, though seldom rich. He had a vein of poetical ore, not of the greatest possible value, but current enough, and he used it liberally on all occasions."

A perusal of the *Records* themselves fully substantiates the justice of these criticisms (26). Over eight hundred pages are filled with anecdotes of incredible triviality, chiefly about second-to fifth-rate celebrities, especially actors and actresses, long since dead and forgotten. The names of Sheridan, Boswell (to whom he suggested a verbal alteration in the title-page of *The Life of*

Johnson), Haydn, Sir Joshua Reynolds, Sir T. Lawrence, Mrs Siddons, Kean, Kemble, raise pleasurable anticipations which are woefully baulked in the sequel. Wordsworth sent him a copy of his *Lyrical Ballads* (published 1798), desiring to know what impression they made upon a man living in the bustle of active life. Byron, acknowledging a present of Taylor's poems, sent four volumes of his own works, with a letter thanking him "for a volume in the good old style of our elders and our betters, which I am very glad to see not yet extinct". In Taylor's private opinion, however, Byron was not sufficiently sublime. It may perhaps be suspected that these transactions exemplify the homage which even poets of nature and great men have been known to pay to the power of the press. The memoirs are constantly hostile to Johnson, whom the author apparently never forgave for the insult to his grandfather's scholarship. He had a poor opinion of Burke, who "did not possess the feelings of a liberal and gentlemanly mind", as was shown by his conduct towards Warren Hastings. He relates how Burke once fished for a compliment on one of his speeches, and received the reply, "Your speech was oppressed by epithet, dislocated by parenthesis, and debilitated by amplification".

A few of his anecdotes are amusing enough. One may be quoted which introduces us to his great-grandfather—the father of the Chevalier. Among his neighbours he had a reputation as a sorcerer, and on one occasion a superstitious countryman invoked his assistance for the recovery of some article which he had lost. Taylor asked him if he had sufficient fortitude to face the devil in order to attain his object. The rustic assured him that he had, whereupon Taylor told him to open a certain drawer. He did so, not without misgivings, and, looking in, exclaimed, "I see nothing but an empty purse". "Well", replied the ancestral Taylor, "and is not that the devil?"

Taylor's one contribution (if it may be so called) to ophthalmic literature, bears the title, *An Address to the Public on Diseases of the Eye, intended chiefly to point out the importance of an early and proper attention in such cases, with remarks on a method lately adopted of treating one of the most frequent Diseases to which the Eye is subject,* etc.(20). This mountain of introduction brings forth a mouse of the most miserable description. Of the new method no details are vouchsafed; evidently application for further information must be made at Hatton Garden. The misery of blindness is illustrated by an apposite quotation from Milton; the necessity of devoting special and unremitting attention to the study of so delicate an organ as the eye, and the author's personal and hereditary qualifications in this respect, are set forth; and the foolish custom of instilling laudanum into inflamed eyes, as practised by "a reputable gentleman in the city", is severely reprobated.

Much the most celebrated of Taylor's poetical works was his *Monsieur Tonson*(22). It relates how a certain wag, Tom King, conceived the idea of knocking every night at the door of an unfortunate refugee in Seven Dials and asking whether "Mr Thompson" lived there; to which the Frenchman replied in a crescendo of remonstrance, "No, Sare; no Monsieur Tonson loges here"; till finally he was driven from hearth and home. At the end of six years he ventured to return, but by pure coincidence it chanced that Tom King, after long absence, was strolling that very night in Seven Dials. Just to see what would happen he once more knocked on the familiar door; the Frenchman appeared, uttered a despairing shriek, "Begar, here's Monsieur Tonson come again!" and fled from the scene for ever.

This not very profound specimen of wit enjoyed a considerable vogue. It was recited with much applause by a Mr Fawcet at the Freemason's Tavern; a dramatised and expanded version was played in 1821 at Drury Lane. It was published first as an undated separate brochure; next in the author's collected poems in 1811 and 1827; then in a collection of *Facetiae*, illustrated by George Cruikshank, in 1830; and finally, in separate form, with Cruikshank's illustrations, in the same year. In the *Sketches by Boz* (chap. v), Dickens refers to Seven Dials as having been "immortalised by Tom King and the Frenchman".

In his other poetical works Taylor undeniably displays a considerable talent for turning out smooth rhythms, but without a trace of the sacred spark which distinguishes poetry from verse. His earliest collection of poems, especially *Verses on Various Occasions* (1795), is full of the stock phrases of the poetaster; Shakespeare is the "bard rever'd", love "hast proudly triumphed o'er my captive soul", his lady-love may "Unbounded empire o'er my breast assume", and so on(21).

His next publication, *The Caledonian Comet* (1810), is an attack on Scott's "magic trash, and Border frays"(23). Of the descriptions of natural scenery he complains that

> Places in this work appear
> As in a Map or Gazetteer.

Scott was much too large of soul to harbour any resentment against his critic, and when Taylor, in financial difficulties, published his collected works by subscription, his name appears in the list of subscribers. Taylor on his side made the *amende honorable* by omitting the offending poem and by the following sonnet. The "higher flight" which thus corrects the faults of the "Lay of the Last Minstrel" is the "Vision of Don Roderick":

> Bard of the North! who wont with strange delight,
> On legends rude of ruffian chiefs to pore
> And form thy lays by ditties quaint of yore,
> That well might perish in oblivion's night,
> Since thou has ventur'd on a higher flight,
> In realms of genuine poetry to soar,
> He greets thee now who dar'd rebuke before,
> Assured thy muse could reach a nobler height.
> Hadst thou first struck the Lusitanian lyre,
> He 'gainst thee ne'er had raised a hostile hand,
> But joy'd to guard thy wreaths from envious ire;
> And glad he sees thee take thy rightful stand;
> For none with purer zeal thy powers admire
> High on the roll with Britain's tuneful band.

The above is quoted as a sufficiently characteristic specimen of the mediocre facility of Taylor's versification and thought. How

bad they could be may be illustrated by the following extract
from a poem on music. Apollo is the giver:

> To Germany then he gave Handel sublime,
> Whose strains will be heard till the death of old Time,
> Those strains that, resistless, pathetic, and grand,
> Comprise the whole scope of the voice and the band.

In 1811 Taylor published his second collection, *Poems on Several
Occasions*(24), the term "Poems" being substituted for the
"Verses" of the earlier volume in deference to the too partial
opinion of his friends. The volume certainly shows an advance in
technique. Many prologues and epilogues written for Mrs Siddons, etc., evince his interest in the drama; the rest of the collection consists of sonnets, tales in the style of "Monsieur Tonson",
imitations of Horace, Gray's "Elegy" (the latter rather good),
and various odds and ends.

The final and complete edition of his works, *Poems on Various
Subjects*(25), published by subscription in two volumes in 1827,
contains a number of new poems of a similar type, and also a
translation of the Odes of Anacreon.

It is only very rarely that Taylor suffers professional matters
to profane the sanctity of his muse. Even in his verses "To a
Lady who had lost an Eye" he manfully resists temptation. On one
occasion, however, perhaps referring to the same lady, he cannot
forgo the opportunity of having a thrust at general surgeons who
pretend to a knowledge of ophthalmology, and of indicating the
spot in Hatton Garden where the milk of the pure doctrine may
be imbibed. On hearing a report that the late Duchess of Devonshire had been deprived of an eye, Venus thus addresses Phoebus:

> Why didst thou not the Dame persuade
> At once to fly to those for aid,
> And Fame declares that such there are*
> Who make THE EYE their fav'rite care.
> For such perchance had soon restor'd
> The radiance that the world ador'd.

---

* The author has no hesitation in saying that he here alludes to his brother, who
is oculist to his Majesty and the Prince of Wales, as well as a Member of the College

To which Phoebus replies:

> Yes *Venus*, had the luckless Dame
> Applied to those who boast the fame
> Of long hereditary skill
> To mitigate each visual ill . . .
> She might have 'scaped the dire event
> That now so deeply we lament.

Her Grace, however, insisted on calling in the popular surgeons.

> Possess'd they are of sense and knowledge
> And sanction'd by the Hall and College.

But

> Though able in their gen'ral art,
> Haply unpractised in a part,
> That nicer part, the wondrous ball,
> Of human powers transcending all. . . .
> Not one is either Knave or Fool,
> They went exact by written rule,
> Hence nothing should I do to smart 'em—
> THE EYE was lost SECUNDUM ARTEM.

Evidently in the grandson many of the traits of the grandfather reappeared, but all on an inferior scale. There is something of the same showiness, the same social disposition, the same itch for writing, though directed to a different end. One pictures a superficial, talkative busybody, flitting from dinner-table to dinner-table with his inexhaustible stock of anecdotes and puns, which might pass muster well enough in a convivial company, but certainly do not stand the cold permanence of print.

BIBLIOGRAPHY AND REFERENCES

I. JOHN TAYLOR, JR.

Works

(1) OLDYS, W. (in collaboration with Taylor). Observations on the Cure of William Taylor, the Blind Boy of Ightham, in Kent; Who being of Surgeons, and who certainly has had the advantage of longer and more varied experience, besides what he derived from parental instruction, than any other practitioner, most probably, in Europe.

born with Cataracts in both Eyes, was at Eight Years of Age, brought to Sight on the 8th of October, 1751, By Mr John Taylor, Junr., Oculist, in Hatton Garden. Containing his strange Notions of Objects upon the first Enjoyment of his new Sense: Also, some Attestations thereof, in a letter written by his Father, Mr William Taylor, Farmer, in the same Parish. Interspers'd with several curious Examples and Remarks, historical and philosophical, thereupon. Dedicated to Dr Monsey, Physician to the Royal Hospital at Chelsea. Also some Address to the Publick, for a Contribution towards the Foundation of an Hospital for the Blind, already begun by some Noble Personages. Printed by E. Owen; in Hand Court, Holborn, 1753.

References

(2) GENTLEMAN'S MAGAZINE. 1787, vol. II, p. 841.

(3) PUBLIC ADVERTISER. December 5th, 1761.

(4) TAYLOR, The Chevalier. History of Travels and Adventures. Vol. III, p. 418, 1761.

(5) WORLIGE, THOS. Print of W. Taylor, Blind boy of Ightham. In British Museum. (See also Reference (26).)

II. RESTORATION OF SIGHT IN THE CONGENITALLY BLIND

(6) MORE, SIR THOMAS. A Dialogue of Syr Thomas More, Knyghte: one of the Counsaill of our souerayne Lord the Kinge, and Chauncellour of his Duchy of Lancaster. Wherin be treatyd diuers maters, as of the veneracion & worship of ymages and relyques praying to saintes, and goyng on pylgrimage. With many other thinges touchyng the pestilent secte of Luther and Tyndale, by the tone bygone in Saxony, and by the tother labored to be brought into England. Made in the yere of our lord 1528. (Bk. I, chap. xiv.)

(7) SHAKESPEARE. Henry VI, Pt. II. Act II, Sc. i.

(8) LOCKE, W. Essay concerning the Human Understanding. 1690. (Bk. II, chap. IX, Sect. 8.)

(9) BERKELEY, GEO. Essay towards a new Theory of Vision. 1709. (xli, lxxix, xcii to cxx, cxxxiii to cxxxv.)

(10) TATLER. No. 55, August 1709.

(11) A Full and True Account of a Miraculous Cure, of a Young Man in Newington, that was Born Blind, and was in Five Minutes brought to Perfect Sight. By Mr Roger Grant, Oculist. London: Printed for Timothy Childe, at the White Hart, at the West End of St Paul's Church yard 1709. Price 2 Pence.

(12) DAILY COURANT. July 30th, 1709.

(13) BRITISH APOLLO. August 5th, August 10th, 1709; January 20th, 1710.

(14) CHESELDEN, W. Phil. Trans. No. 402, p. 447, 1728.

(15) SMITH, R. A compleat System of Opticks. Cambridge, 1738. Bk. I, chap. V, p. 42. (Quotation of another paper by Cheselden.) Also p. 27.

(16) HIRSCHBERG, J. Graefe-Saemisch Handbuch d. ges. Augenheilk. 1911. II Theil, XIV Bd. xxiii Kap. 3 Buch, II Theil, p. 404. XIII Bd. 3 Buch, p. 453, 1908. (See also References (1) and (5).)

III. ROGER GRANT

(17) SPECTATOR. No. 444, July 30th, 1712; No. 472, September 1st, 1712; No. 547, November 27th, 1712.

(18) FOLIO SHEET. 1830. C. 1 (18) in British Museum.

(19) BRITISH APOLLO. 1709 *et seq. passim.* (See also References (10), (11), (12), (13).)

IV. JOHN TAYLOR, TERTIUS

Works

(20) An Address to the Public on Diseases of the Eye, intended chiefly to point out the importance of an early and proper attention in such cases, with remarks on a method lately adopted of treating one of the most frequent Diseases to which the Eye is subject. By J. Taylor, Oculist to His Majesty; M.D. of the University of Basle; Member of the Helvetic Physico-Medical Society; the Corporation of Surgeons of London, &c., &c. Qui dat videre, dat vivere. Cic. London: Printed for the Author; and to be had gratis at his House in the Adelphi. MDCCXCIV.

(21) Verses on Various Occasions. "I left no calling for this idle trade." London. Printed by B. M. Millan, Printer to His Royal Highness the Prince of Wales; Sold by J. Debrett, Piccadilly; and Cullen & Co., Pall Mall. M. DCC. XCV.

(22) Monsieur Tonson, a Tale, written by Mr Taylor, and recited in London by Mr Fawcet, to crowded audiences with universal applause. Glasgow: Printed for and sold by Brash & Read.

Published again in collection of *Facetiae* illustrated by Geo. Cruikshank. London: A. Miller, and Constable & Co., Edinburgh. 1830. Same edition separately printed in same year. Price 1s. Published also in collected poems of 1811 and 1827.

(23) The Caledonian Comet.

"I had rather be a kitten, and cry Mew,
    Than one of these same metre Ballad-mongers."
"A clip-wing'd griffin, and a moulten raven—
    And such a deal of skimble-skamble stuff."

London: Printed for W. Dwyer, 29, Holborn Hill. 1810.

(24) Poems on Several Occasions: consisting of sonnets, miscellaneous pieces, prologues and epilogues,—tales, imitations, etc. Edinburgh: Printed by George Ramsay and Company, for John Murray, London, and Archibald Constable & Co., Edinburgh. 1811.

(25) Poems on Various Subjects by John Taylor, Esq. "Dear Sir, I have to thank you for a volume written in the good old style of our Elders and our Betters, which I am very glad to see is not yet extinct." Extract from a letter from the late Lord Byron to the Author. In two Volumes. Vol. 1. London. Printed for Payne & Foss, Pall Mall; Longman, Rees, Orme & Co., Paternoster Row; J. Richardson, Royal Exchange; and J. Murray, Albemarle Street. 1827.

(26) Records of my Life; by the late John Taylor, Esquire, Author of "Monsieur Tonson". In two volumes. Vol. 1. London: Edward Bull, Holles Street, 1832.

Reference

(27) GENTLEMAN'S MAGAZINE. 1832, vol. CII, ii, p. 542; 1826, vol. XCVI, ii, p. 158. Individual poems also published in Gentleman's Magazine for many years before his death.

APPENDIX

Sloane MS. 75 fol. 145

DE CURA OCULORUM

COLLIRIUM oculis egris sive fuerit ex percussione sive humoribus ibidem concurrentibus sic fiet / Recipe albuminem ovi crudi et bene despumetur cui vero addatur medietatem aque rosacee et tantundem lactis femine quibus addatur de Croci qui pondus unius denarii vel obuli et resolvatur in predicto liquore. Tunc de predicto liquore imponatur due gutte vel (? tres) et in oculo. Fiat emplastrum de stupis lini mundis et delicatis in predicto liquore bene madefactis in quo emplastro ponatur Crocus predictus et immediate super oculum ponatur. Istud multa prefecit juvamenta dolorem mitigat et sanguinem mundificat et mollificat et desiccacionem uneo humiectat clara ovi primo mitigat que super suavis est /

Constringit humores ne ad oculos currant et humores oculorum naturales custodit ne dissolvantur.

Purificat et nullam superfluitatem aliorum humorum neque spumum ad oculos venire permittit et sanat / Et clara ovi que clarificat oculum nam est ejusdem qualitatis cum oculo. Crocus roborem oculorum ex sanguine abstringit et fluxum humorum ad oculum prohibet panum qua maculam oculorum delet est enim resolutinum et macritatinum cum quadem stiptificate (*sic*).

Aqua Rosarum calorem naturalem in oculo abterat et reprimerit cerebrum que confortat et species animales multiplicat et multa alia comoda facit. Cum hac medicina quae plures horribiliter lesos in oculis proficere curavi cum ea vero curavi quandam cujus oculus cum gladio percussus super genam pendebat ad grossiciem unius ovi qui postea cum eodem oculo satis bene vidit.

2. Et quum predictum emplastrum dessiccatum fuerit reponatur iterum in predicto liquore et cum mollificatum fuerit ad oculum ponatur. Iterum si oculus percussus fere fuerit erectus et valde sanguineolentus succus lappe inverse id est Agrimonie cum albumine ovi dispumati commisseatur et cum stupis lini deforis apponatur et bene sanabitur pro certo / Idem succus facit foliorum Sambuci

predicto meo paratus Ut de Agrimonie dictum est sepius idem probavi et si predictus addatur Crocus efficiacior erit medicina // Inflacionem et emiciam palpebrarum vel oculorum causa melancolie / Facta prius purgatione cum pillulis sine quibus esse nolo ponatur istud emplastrum. Recipe pomum acerbum et sub cinere coctum a cortice qua mandatum ad iiii poma additur clara unius ovi et folium pistentur Et de isto emplastro cum stupis lini bis in die oculo clauso appone / Istud emplastrum primo detumescit oculum.

In proprio loco collocat. 3°. Dolorem mitigat et lumine recuperat secundum Lanifrancum et nota quod si patiens juvenis fuerit multum ei comperet fleabotomari de vena in medio frontis antequam purgetur cum predictis pillulis Psillium in aquam frigidam infusum cum tota muscilagine apponatur oculis qua eorum forte incendium summe valet.

Ruborem omnem oculorum et puritum palpebre delet Collirium rubrorum quod sit de cujus Rubi id est *Redebrerecropys* ad modum salse bene tritis et in vino albo decoctis ad medietatem totius. Quo facto calor et usui reserva scilicet autem istam caram nesciundatur vena frontis /

Item qua ruborem oculorum vinum album decoctionis Aloes epatice in oculo distillatum summum est remedium / Scabiem palpebrarum

3. intus tritum nam bonam carnem optime generat et malam corrodit, nutritur.

(i d) Autem sic licugirum pulverizetur et si subtilliter cui addatur olei rosacei partes 2° et aceti pars una semper movendo donec valde augmentetur et forma unguenti albi recipiat / Istud vero valde rectificat ulcera antiqua calida oculis percussis vel ferro inscisis Apponatur vitellum ovi crudi cum oleo rosarum ad eorum dolorem mitigandum lippitudinem oculorum curat aqua decoctionis rosarum et gallarum videlicet aqua pluvalium si oculi inde alluantur tepide et idem videlicet quam incendium oculorum. Tuthia dessicat sive mordicacione et est utilis olceribus oculorum et fluxui acriti in ipsis et abluta conservat sanitate oculorum si infere in oculis ponatur / Iterum Tuthia nonies ignita fortiter postea quum quinquies extincta in urina pure virginis et quater in aqua rosacea vel vino albo sed in ultima combustione non extinguatur in aliquo liquore sed per se frigescere permittetur. Postea super lapidem molarem subtillissime tritata et per pannum subtillissimum tritonizetur. Postea distemperetur in eodem liquore quo prius fuerit extincta aliqualiter spisse Quo facta Tuthia sic temperata infra pelvem eneum mundissimum et con-

cavum undique circa fundum et latera liniatur. Ita ut non decurrat postea accipiatur bonum aloes epaticum et pulverizetur sed non multum
subtilliter et super carbones lente candentes propiciatur. Quo facto
statim pelvis cum Tuthia inuncta super carbones supina inversetur ut
possit summum aloes recipere et sic jaceat donec id in pelvi dessicatum
fuerit.

Quo facto et in pelvi abradatur et ad solem dessiccetur postea pulverizetur et iterum tritonizetur et usui reservetur pulvis id est. Iste sic
paratus maculam oculorum delet et ruborem ardoremque oculorum
refrigerat et lacrimas stringit quam visum comfortat atque conservat /
vel pars de isto pulvere et parum de auxbugia caponis fieri unguentum
et uti ad predictam remollicius in oculo prius appositis // Vel de sola
Tuthia combusta et ut predicta preparata et ut predicta pulverizata
et post panno lineo subtilli posita et in vino bene tacta Et postquam
infrigida fuerit de illa medicia cum penna una gutta vel 2º instilletur.
Hoc idem lacrimas et ruborem oculorum delet et visum clarificat. /
Istud Tuchia per se solam predicto modo parata et pulverizata et cum
zucare Keffetino ante commixta in oculo infero posita corrodit suaviter
pannum in oculo et maculam lumine quorum oculorum clarificat pal-
pebras tumefactas subtiliat ruborem atque puritum palpebrarum delet
lacrimas que constringit et oculum ampliat visum quod fortificat et
conservat Et hoc probavi. Remolliciam oculorum sunt lac mulieris
calidum et resens impositum / Lac assine / Albumine ovi / Sanguis
columbe de sub ala ejus extractus / Tuchia apud Apothecarios
inventur ad vendendum libra cujus videlicet xii vel xvi^d cujus lanie
tenuissime precipue sunt eligende transfertur de partibus transmarinis.

Secundum Johannes Damascenum in omni dolore oculorum et
contra defectum visus primo considerari oportet sit de causa calida
vel frigida Si de causa calida primo digeratur Materia cum sirupo
acetosa per 3 dies vel 4. Recipe digesta vero maº pro clistere mollifi-
catiam ex decoctione malvarum mane debeo evacuare totum corpus

cum $\frac{I}{I}$l / Electuarius de succo rosarum acuatur cum diag^e

dis et ter secure priores cum localibus remediis operari serv' quas
tui videtur expedire.

(ii) In frigida vero causa primo digeratur mixta cum oximelle
diuretico vel squillitico demi detur clistere ut predictum est mane
purgetur corpus cum ȝ ierapige galieni quod in apoticharia invenietur
et postea ad localia precedatur remedia. Lac mulieris vel asine cum
vitello ovi crudi croco et oleo rosarum ad oculum superpositum satis
mitigat et digerit ignea oculorum aparat et inflationes et si succus Apii

viridis id est *smallache* vel vervuine vel portulace id est purcelane vel
rosarum vel psillii, vel sempervine, id est rubarb, que omnes sunt
repercussive predictis adderetur magis erit mitigative dolorum Nam
quicunque repercuciunt materiam calidam mitigant et ejus fervorem
cum stupe appone // Contingit oculorum incendium forte psillium in
aqua frigida infusum cum bonibace vel stupis lini appone et sanabitur /

Lippitudinem oculorum et lacrimas quamvis propociens senex et de-
crepitus fuerit optime curat hoc unguentum multo enim hoc probavi
Quod sic fit pelvis concavus eneus bene mundatus de butiro resenti
per inferius perunctus sic stet per noctem. mane vero super ollam vel
patellam in quam fit urina hominis acerbam et calescam inversetur
pelvis predictus et sic recipiat summum urine et butirum liquefiat cum
a urina infrigidata fuerit deponatur pelvis et sic stare permittatur per
diem integrum postea abradatur butirum quod viride apparebit et
cum parum de pinguedine caponis ad solem vel ad ignem liquefacto
conmisce et in pixide cerata reconde donec idem opus humeris.
Desiccentur bene palpebre cum panno lineo molli et statim cum
predicto unguento super palmam manus liqueres caute palpebre
inungantur ne in oculis decurrat et clausis oculis cum benda
ligetur et sic iaceat per nocte mane vero dissolvatur scilicet non
abluatur donec sanus fuerit / Iterum vero abluatur cum aqua tepida
sed nullo cum frigida // Et nota pro certo quod frequens ablu-
cione cum urina propria pacientis puritus vel puncturas aquositatem
vel si quia sabulum senserit in oculis et cotidiana debilitatem visus ex
senio inurie iuvat omnia namque nocumenta predicta delet et visum
confortat atque forisficat et conservat et precipue alippitudine // Ista
medicina mimet summe proficiebat cum oculos meos in studendo et
scribendo usque ad annum etatis mee lxx. Multum debilitaverim //
Et sciantur presentes et futuri qui ego Johannes de Ardern cirurgi-
corum minimusque hunc libellum propria manu mea exaravi apud
London anno victorii regni regis Ricardi 2ⁱ primo et etatis mee lxx et
quavis ista medicina videatur esse communis nichilominus cara
habeatur cum innumerabiles tempore meo ex predictis passionibus
cum ea curaverim scit deus quod non meum cōr // Sed est notum
quod urina non debet esse resens sed aliquantulum acerba hoc est
etatis duorum dierum in estate et trium in hieme et si urina fuerit
iniecta in vase ad inunctum usitato tunc in mane sequenti valebit satis
ad predictam qua urina resens gerat vermes in manibus et palpebris si
inde laventur / Cum medicina hac predicta et usu seminis feniculi
poterit homo se a cecitate oculorum et predictis passionibus curare.

(iii d) et preservare sine altera alia medicina ut probavi nisi fuerit peniores regius et dispositionis Et post ablucionem cum urina tunc debat pacientes clausis oculis lavare faciem et oculos cum aqua tepida et cum panno abstergere. Crocus orientalis super tegulam calidam dessicatus et pulverizatus et post cum albumine ovi bene despumato distemperatus et postea quod ex eo clarius est in oculis imponatur / et recluso oculo suppone emplastrum de vitellis ovi crudis cum dicto croco temperatis super stupas lini mundas roborem oculorum ex sanguine et macula aufert mirifice / Balsami naturalis si una gutta vel due gutte in oculo pannum vel maculam habente bis vel ter instilletur oculum de predictis bene mundificat et sine mordicacione violenta et visum fortiter acuit et in naturali virtute preservat et hoc probavi de me ipso et pluribus aliis Quod Balsamum semper habui imprompto. Unguentum laxatum non violentum quia si inde ungatur venter ab umbilico inferiis suaviter ducet ad 4 cellas vel 5 sic confiteor Recipe succum Ebuli et Sambuci et bene cum auxungia porci veteri pistentur sine igne donec succus in auxilia imbibatur: denum addatur pulveris Aloes cicotrici subtilissime pulverizati et bene cum predicta auxungia commisceatur sine igne et fiat unguentum et usui reservetur donec opus de ventrice inferius ab umbilico inferius ungatur et emplastretur Diaflacta qua summe deopilat eparum et specialem quarum valet hydropica epaticis et splenetitis. Fr. Gordon in antidotare suo in lilio Sic fiet. Recipe lacte ℥ vi, Costi spicenarde reubrei Xilobalsami, Cassie Lignei Cynamoni, Assari, Croci, Squinanti, Masticis, Aristologie, rotunde et longe, Mirrhe, Gentiane, Maratri, Apii, diversis gariofilis, folii Cumini, Eupatori, Nucis Muscate, Absinthii, Cardamoni, Cucube, aliena ℥ ij, pulverizatur et cum zucare dentur, de isto coclearum plenum vino rubeo calescone Ista receptione continiet uncias et ℥ ij et ℥ super medicamen que valet in acutis et contra epacis calorem et contra sitim.

Recipe Rosarum ℥ vi spodii seminis Portulaci seminis fundorum mundatorum succi liquirice aliam ℥ ij amid' draganti aliam ℥ i et ℥ in zucari, $\frac{I}{i}$ s' Camphor ℥ i fiant trocisti cum muscilagine Psilli et teneantur in ore donec per se dissolvantur et paulatim transgluciantur / Ita recipe continet $\frac{I}{i}$ et ℥ ij Trocisti de spodio probatur quam calorem epatis et tussim siccam et consumpciones corporis qui cognoscitur propriam communes musculorum brachiorum et manus / Recipe Rosarum $\frac{I}{i}$ et

℥ iij zucari spodii succi liquiricii aliam ℥t u' omne sandale Portulace, Endivie, aliam Scrupulos iii, Melonis, Cucumeris, et Cucurbite, another ℥ i Tempora cum muscilagine Psilii et da cum sirupo Violarum, / Medicamen purgans humores calidos ad epate / Recipe Reubri

℥ i̅ lacte Rosarum spodii Absinthii, Eupatoris, Squinanti, aliam ℥ i

Confice cum succo Endivie fiant in trocisti et cum uti volueris dentur cum aqua decoccionis Endivie vel cum aqua ejusdem vel Scariole Iterum trissera Saracenica Multim vz in hoc casu.

GENERAL INDEX

Printed in the United States
By Bookmasters